PERMANENT WEIGHT LOSS

The Self-Nurtuing Mindset,
the Habits, and the Diet Strategy
for Genuine, Lasting Change

by Scott Abel

Published by:

Scott Abel

© Copyright 2016 – Scott Abel

ISBN-13: 978-1530645084
ISBN-10: 1530645085

ALL RIGHTS RESERVED. No part of this publication may be reproduced or transmitted in any form whatsoever, electronic, or mechanical, including photocopying, recording, or by any informational storage or retrieval system without express written, dated and signed permission from the author.

Table of Contents

Introduction 7

Chapter 1. It's Time To Get Real About Getting Real 31

Chapter 2. An Integrated Approach to Fitness 43

Chapter 3. The Self-Nurturing Mindset 59

Chapter 4. Mindfulness and the Buddhist Approach to End Suffering 71

Chapter 5. Karl Albrecht's Four Mental Habits to Increase Productivity 99

Chapter 6. The Diet Strategy Mindset 119

Practical Section:

Getting Started 139

Your Diet Strategy and Meal Plan 145

Your Exercise Plan 169

Self-Investigation Section 193

About the Author

Scott Abel has been involved in the diet, fitness, and bodybuilding industries for over four decades. He has written for, or been featured in magazines like *Muscle & Fitness*, *Flex*, *Muscle Mag*, *T-Nation*, and many more.

In recent years he has focused on lasting, permanent change, and on providing a realistic, practical perspective on fitness.

He blogs at scottabelfitness.com/blog. At his website, scottabelfitness.com, you can also download two free books: *Introduction to Metabolic Enhancement Training*, and *The Mindset of Achievement*.

Introduction

Greg is in his early fifties. He is divorced and working middle management at a large company. He's 5'10" and very overweight at around 280 lbs. He desperately wants to diet down and reach a healthy weight.

Greg tells me he constantly tries to diet, lasts a few days at most, and then quits. Every morning he wakes up and tells himself that this will finally be the day he gets it all together. But he never does, and this drives him nuts. He always finds a reason to eat more than he had planned to, or he ignores his plans entirely. At one point he even signed up for a service that delivered meals to his house, but he had the same problem—finding reasons to eat a bit more here and there, or ignoring the pre-made meal plan entirely.

Every day, by lunchtime, he's very hungry, and he usually eats out with coworkers who are also overweight. He comes home from work and feels guilty that another day has gone by, and yet again he hasn't made a real attempt at dieting. He looks into an empty fridge and vows to shop for groceries this weekend. He orders delivery and eats alone. When he writes me to tell me all this, he also wants to know how long it would take me to write a new, custom diet to follow. He doesn't want actual coaching or anything. He just wants the diet.

Sylvia has written me several times over the years, though she has never hired me for coaching. She is about 5'3" and, to her frustration, her weight has been climbing over the years so that she is now closing in on 185 lbs. Understandably, she wants to do something about it.

She works a full-time job. She has three kids at home, and she stays in a very unhappy and unsatisfying marriage because of her kids. She's only in her forties, but she looks much older. She says she hardly ever smiles and really, truly means it. She's sleep deprived, too. Sometimes this is through no fault of her own, but often it is just from not going to bed at a reasonable hour, even when she had the chance. She doesn't see this as being connected to her climbing weight. Whenever she gets stressed, angry, or frustrated—which seems to her to be "all the time" now—she has some wine, or she snacks. Sometimes she'll get fed up and go on a crash diet, lose some weight, then gain it all back. Finally, she'll write me again and ask me what she's doing wrong. "Which diet is right for me?" she wants to know. The last time she wrote, she said what she thought she really needed was a diet to "speed up her metabolism."

Like Greg, Sylvia continues to think that "a diet" will solve her weight problem. But here's the truth: it's not the diet.

Jennifer isn't 30 yet and she writes me because some day she dreams of competing in a figure competition or a bikini contest. She's not obese, but she does have a good 40-50 lbs. to lose, she says. She is looking for a program to get her "tight abs and tight glutes." However, by her own admission, she is "sporadic at best" when it comes to consistency, with both diet and exercise. Because of this, she is thinking of going low carb for a while, and she wants to know my opinion on that. She's also considering doing a nine-day cleanse that some of her friends are doing.

Jennifer says she struggles with low self-esteem and feelings of inadequacy. She is worried about what other people say about her or are thinking about her. She thinks if she could just drop this weight and compete, it would set her on a more permanent path to health and wellness. She thinks her self-esteem issues and anxiety issues will be solved if she could just find the right diet and sculpt a better body. She doesn't see that it's the other way around: these very issues will block her from the consistency she's after, and they'll block her from achieving a better body.

Do you see yourself in any of the examples above?

I've changed the names, but all of the above examples are from real people who write me looking for help. What they have in common is a certain level of self-deception. The weight issues are a reflection of issues that go deeper than what diet someone is on.

Many, many people write to me looking for a diet as a solution to problems that a diet by itself cannot solve. Even with the right diet, or the so-called "perfect" meal plan, many people are not mentally or emotionally ready to use a diet properly in a sustainable way.

Certain levels of mental and emotional fitness must be established before weight loss and physique transformation can be successfully undertaken for long-term results.

As you will learn in this project, weight loss

and consistency are by-products of something much greater. Without the right mindset in place, a diet becomes a pressure-filled "have to" process of self-measuring and self-judging that just gets worse and worse. But when the proper mindset *is* in place, everything else will fall into place as well.

To explain what I mean, let's look at the other side of the spectrum.

Susan first came to me when I ran on online course on women's eating, food, and body image issues. So many elements of the course struck a chord with her that she knew she had to sign up for the one-on-one coaching. In the initial stages of our working together, we focused only on how she thought and felt around food, and how she felt and thought about dieting and herself. We put a diet strategy in place initially just as a "guideline" for healthy eating. At first, she rebelled against not having someone like me serving as her food police. However, together we worked on her integrated fitness and her emotional wellness. We kept going. So far she has lost 35 lbs., and I can tell from her regular coaching check-ins that she will continue to lose the weight. I have no doubt she will keep it off. She's in a much better place mentally. The food and diet are beginning to take care of themselves. She doesn't jump from one diet to the next. She follows simple guidelines as part of a reasonable diet strategy, but then she moves on with her very busy life.

Similarly, JP came to me overweight. He had been unsuccessful at previous attempts at dieting and getting in shape, and he knew it was time to get real. Instead of trying more and more diets, he hired a coach. He followed me online and used the respect he had for me as motivation to "not let me down." As his coach, I used this aspect of JP's psyche to ensure that he wouldn't let himself down. He didn't. Not by a long shot!

JP now works entirely on his own "right mind" solution to honour any of the physique commitments he makes to himself. (I will talk more about "right mind" later on.) He is such a model client that I have written about him several times in my books and on my blog.

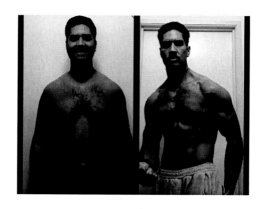

Finally, Shawn has been with me as a client for years. He is formerly obese, and now he works as a personal trainer in one of the most respected facilities in his area. He enjoys working out and golfing. One of Shawn's initial weight-loss challenges was to get rid of the rather intimidating idea that he'd never get to eat his favourite foods again. Shawn would aim for perfection, but the idea that he'd never enjoy certain foods ever again would always make him subconsciously rebel against whatever diet he was on. We spent some time training Shawn's metabolism with a simple whole foods diet, and when his metabolism and his head were ready, we got Shawn on my Cycle Diet. He now enjoys weekly cheat days and takes a week off-diet and working out for vacations and other special events.

Shawn maintains his weight loss, but still gets to enjoy his favourite foods. His diet strategy is a part of his lifestyle, and nothing more. Before, he was trying to lose weight by making his diet his whole life. Now has proper perspective. He has lost well over 100 lbs. and has kept that weight off for years. He did it by getting real, and by taking an integrative approach to his fitness and wellness. His remarkable weight loss was a by-product of a larger commitment he had made to himself.

Alba is another client who, like JP, has been featured on my blog. She was also a former student in the same women's eating and food issues course as Susan, above. She is a very busy mom, and she had a previous EDNOS issue (Eating Disorder Not Otherwise Specified). She was using food for emotional comfort and stability. Before we worked together, she thought dieting and losing weight would be her solution, and that these things would help her feel better about herself. She learned that "getting real" meant it was actually the other way around: feeling better about herself would help her to eat healthier and want to take better care of herself.

As we worked together, she realized that her food and weight issues were mindset issues. By working on herself from the inside out, she has not only lost weight, but she looks decades younger, too! We worked on Alba's mindset more than we ever focused on policing her diet. In fact, once she learned that her coach was never going to judge her but was always there to support her, she was able to do the same for herself. She stopped judging herself and started supporting and nurturing both herself and her body. She has recently joined a gym (we started with a training program she could do at home) and she can't even remember why she was previously so deathly afraid of going to one.

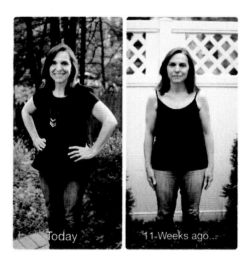

What all of these successful clients have in common is more than just soliciting the help of a coach. In fact, I would say that seeking a coach part was actually a sign of something *else*. It's a sign that they were willing to make a real change, and they were willing to do it on change's terms. Many people want change, but only on their own terms, so they try the same things again and again.

The successful clients you just read about were able to see their weight issues in new ways, and they learned it was about more than just their weight. This helped them to develop "right mindfulness," which you will read and learn about later. Eventually, their "right mindfulness" led to "right intention," "right action," and "right living." These clients let go of the battle mindset and instead developed a mindset that was more self-nurturing and self-motivating.

You don't need to hire a coach to do this. But you do need to get real about taking a truly integrative approach to fitness, and you need to let go of the diet-mentality madness, once and for all.

The rest of this project is about walking you through this change. Part of this can be done just by reading and absorbing this book, but part of it will only come when you get to the practical section. I've included self-investigation questions and exercises at the very end, and I've also included sustainable diet strategies and exercise suggestions.

However, a warning: if you skip to the example meal plans, or you read this stuff but don't actually follow through on *any* of the exercises, then not much is likely to change for you. You can skip to the diet or exercises, but until you take the inside-out approach, they just won't work. Remember, even the "right diet" won't work until you're ready for it.

There is an old expression in Eastern philosophy:

"Before enlightenment, I chopped wood and carried water; after enlightenment, I chopped wood and carried water."

Listen, to lose weight you will have to control your diet and commit to a sound and healthy diet strategy. Of course that's true. You will have to be consistent with a regular exercise program. That remains true as well.

To echo the saying above, you still chop wood and carry water, as it were, but after you get into the right mindset, you will approach these things from a totally different place. It's a place based on self-awareness, not self-delusion. It is a place focused on self-nurturing and on calm, patient energy. From this place, you'll be able to tune out or ignore thoughts of self-rejection, and you'll be able to avoid constant self-measurement and self-judging.

No worthwhile journey is going to be easy. This is especially true at first, when everything is new.

If you've tried dieting in the past, or you identify with any of the people above (even the successful ones), there will be a lot of back and forth between the faulty mindset of the North American diet mentality and the new mindfulness mindset that you will use to finally lose weight and keep it off.

The process will be different for each of you. Many emotions will come to the surface. There will be a lot of back and forth as your current mindset will always want to take over. As the saying goes, "It takes a habit to break a habit."

Like anything else, the more you practice this stuff, the better you will become. If you just read it all and expect magic to somehow just happen, you aren't getting real about the change you want.

Here's the thing: it has always been up to you. The real solution has never been in outside forces like diets or pills or cleanses. The solution is inside you, right now.

Embracing Change

If you are someone with substantial weight to lose, chances are you have already been on at least one, and likely more than a few, fad diets. The thought of doing something different may be intimidating, to say the least. You may think that without a specific diet to follow, you will be bigger than ever.

First, you need to remind yourself that following "diets" has never led you to long-term, sustainable, and substantial weight loss or you wouldn't be reading this book.

Second, it is still perfectly okay to embrace a certain amount of routine and regimentation. I even recommend that, and I will talk more about it later. But what you'll find is that there is a world of difference between arbitrary outside-in rules that you "have to" follow, and making your own, empowered choices about your eating routine and lifestyle.

Substantial weight loss can only be accomplished and sustained by developing a lifestyle and a mindset that supports it. Yes, you can employ a diet strategy, but that's different from "a diet," as I hope the rest of this book will show.

I realize that when you're just starting out, all this mindset stuff sounds great and all, but really all you want is to lose this excess weight. To that I would say, consider the old Buddhist expression: "You can get there; you just have to stop trying so hard." It seems counterintuitive, but you need to trust that this is the fastest way to get from A to B.

This means taking the focus off of what you want and putting the focus on the process that takes you there. You need a lifestyle habit, and when you develop that, you aren't expending so much useless "willpower energy" to lose weight.

It just becomes how you choose to live.

You have to embrace that the solution is **within you**. This is true **mentally, emotionally,** and **behaviourally**. All three of these realms must be on the same page in order for you to get to where you want to be. When that happens, each of the three realms support and mutually reinforce one another. For example, issues in the emotional realm are easier to deal with if the mental and behavioural realms are there for you to lean on.

Like so many others who struggle with weight issues, you probably already have a decent idea of what you have to do to achieve your substantial weight loss goal. In a general way, this usually gets whittled down to something like, "Eat less, move more." (I would also add, "Don't go to extremes.")

Yet you haven't done it yet.

Why?

The answer, I would argue, is because you are not properly taking care of all three realms. You're not taking the integrated approach. "Eat less, move more," *seems* to concern only the behavioural realm. But that's an illusion. As I said, all three realms are there to reinforce and support one another.

Most diets, and most fitness industry competitions and so on, promise that if you change the behaviour, the mind and emotions just sort of follow along. This is the implicit message on so many supplement ads and infomercial testimonials. They promise that you can diet your way to a better, happier life. They promise that if you follow their special secret diet and exercise rules (which are totally different and unique and unlike all those *other* diet rules), then your mind will follow suit.

That's too simple. Take an integrated approach. Pay attention to the mind and your mental realm. Pay attention and be aware of your emotions. The behaviour—that is, following the diet—is still there for you to do, but it's much easier. I repeat: quality of mindset determines quality of behaviour. Or, as you will see, "right mind" leads to "right action" because of "right intention."

Mindset and Behaviour

William James, often referred to as the father of modern psychology, said, "The greatest discovery of my generation is that human beings, by changing the inner attitudes of their minds, can change the outer aspects of their lives. […] It is so unfortunate that more people will not accept this tremendous discovery and begin living it."

This is why I am telling you that if you have substantial weight to lose, and if you truly want to both lose it and keep it off, that process must begin in your mind. For example, let's say you "follow a diet" exactly as you should. It seems like you have taken care of the behaviour part, right? But if the behaviour is tainted by a bad mindset—one steeped in how hard and horrible all this dieting and exercise is, combined with an ongoing sense of struggle and the fact that you "have to" follow all these absurd rules—then the behaviour won't last long.

I repeat: quality of mindset determines quality of behaviour.

Consider the alternate approach, where you've got an empowered mindset towards your behaviours.

You follow a set of reasonable guidelines. You don't think of it as suffering. When you make a meal you don't see it as something you "have" to do but as something you have chosen to do, and as something that takes you closer to your goals. You feel good about what you're doing. How much longer will that behaviour last? If you have the right mindset, it can go on indefinitely.

All this gets reinforced when you add in the fact that a proper and grounded mindset will prevent you from indulging in panicked, desperate behaviours like cutting out all carbs or only eating 400 calories a day for the next week.

Consistently self-directing your mind is the first step to losing substantial weight and keeping it off. Self-directing your mind simply means taking time to examine thoughts as they come into your head. Then you can assess whether these thoughts are true and whether they help you or hurt you.

You can direct your mind what to think about and how to think about it. Most people have left their mindset on "default." You have to self-direct your mind away from all this stinkin' thinkin' about end results. You have to self-direct your mind towards experiencing and embracing the process: making your meals, getting proper sleep, staying consistent without getting sidetracked by empty promises on the covers of magazines.

I still do this myself. Every day, the second I wake up, I sit on the edge of my bed and say a gratitude prayer, and then I mentally direct my mind about what I have to do in the next several minutes and the next several hours. Maybe it's organizing my notes for this project, maybe it's answering client emails first. I aim to focus on the process.

I enjoy doing this because, when I do it, I find there is less room for distraction. You will find this, as well, once you start practicing this self-directing mindset.

(You'll also find that although self-directing your mind technically takes place in the *mental* realm, if you do it each day as soon as you wake up, then isn't it also, in some sense, a habitual *behaviour*? Moreover, when I do it, I feel better *emotionally*, too, because I'm focusing on what I need to, and frankly, that just plain feels good. Again, these three realms overlap and support one another.)

I've had so many clients succeed just by reframing their thoughts with self-direction. One client who was a former binge eater had a dream where she binged, even though she hadn't done so in months and months. When she woke up she reminded herself that this was simply her subconscious mind's way of reminding her conscious mind to "stay responsible." I thought that was an amazing way to frame it. She self-directed her mind towards thoughts and behaviours that would serve her during the day ahead. She used a subconscious experience as a way to reframe and then direct her thoughts away from what she doesn't want and towards what she *needs to do*.

I had another client who just wrote me this morning. He was at a party and there were nachos, as well as his favourite dessert. His old mindset kicked in, and he wanted to have that dessert "so badly." Then he stopped himself right there by addressing his thoughts.

He said to himself, "Here I go again. I want to lose weight, but I want nachos and cake the second I see them. Where has fighting these urges ever got me in the past? How is this old way of thinking ever going to get me anywhere, other than where it always got me before? Screw that. I've got better things to think about. I've had enough cake and nachos for a lifetime. They're not going to taste any different. This isn't about what I want to do; this is what I need to do when the challenge is presented."

Then he told me he used a trick I'd told him about previously. He told his mind to just "change the channel." He asked himself if this level of thinking was taking care of himself in a healthy way. The answer was no, so he changed the channel. He directed his mind to thinking about his workout for tomorrow and how that was going to feel. He started thinking about needing to do his food prep later this week. He changed the channel away from the mindset of resistance (standing there, looking at the food, trying to resist his urge to indulge) and he self-directed his thoughts "towards" the process of what he needs to do to stay true to doing what it takes. Sometimes it can be that simple.

He also asked his body what it wanted and needed from him. It didn't *need* a bunch of nachos and cake. This is also part of him "changing the channel" mentally. Your body is always communicating with you. Your body's authentic message is, "Nurture me and take care of me. I'm trying to take care of you. I'm trying to work with you. Please work with me, as well. Don't work 'on' me."

Dr. Christine Northrup said, "Changes that are nurtured into being are more likely to be permanent." That is what this project is about. Trying to starve yourself or beat your body into submission, trying to self-hate your way to permanent weight loss, trying to fight against what you don't want—none of this is going to work.

You are unique. Any blocks you have to progress are more than likely unique to you. That uniqueness, moreover, is likely in your mind, not your physiology. How you think and feel based on the life you have lived, that is unique to you.

But what you think about, and how you think about what you think about—that is within your control.

The mistake is setting out to lose substantial weight in order to reform your whole life. I've had several clients who were trying to lose weight and get in shape "for their spouse." As long as that was the reason they were trying to lose weight, they could never do it. They had to find a truer, more authentic source of motivation. It can't be external. It has to come from within.

Ironically, in one instance, while we were working on my client's source of motivation, her relationship with her spouse ended very suddenly. What do you think happened? She was able to lose weight and get in remarkable shape. She was motivated to do it for herself and not for someone else. That other person judging what they ate all the time was no longer there, so the pressure was gone. She found a more authentic source of motivation.

All the stress and obsession we have about our weight is often what weighs heaviest upon us. Our culture is one that body shames relentlessly, making the problem even worse. This creates a lot of mental and emotional baggage (to say the least), so that before you can deal with the actual, physical weight, you have to deal with the stuff inside.

We need to change our thinking about self-worth, self-respect, and self-acceptance, and we need to use self-nurturing to get there.

Your self-worth is not something you have to prove to the world by losing a lot of weight or something.

You are already worthy. Your self-worth should be a given. It is something no one can take away from you.

When your self-worth is already a given, self-nurturing your way to being more productive is easier. When self-worth is a given, then the idea of self-hating your way towards anything is revealed for what it has always been: absurd.

A good way to begin all of this is by starting with a simple command I once heard in a seminar. As with dog obedience training, the first three commands are, "Sit, stay, and heal." (Note the spelling of "heal"!)

It's all about fostering calm, peaceful, self-connected energy. Sometimes, to foster this kind of energy, you have to "sit" and "stay" right where you are and do nothing. Healing begins from there, and healthy change begins from there.

Losing a substantial amount of weight is a

long-term process. Learn to "sit" with your thoughts, "stay" with the self-nurturing process, and then just let yourself "heal." You are allowed to want to change this or that aspect of your body, especially if you think it is unhealthy. But you need to do so with a positive, self-nurturing energy and attitude.

Chapter 1.
It's Time To Get Real About Getting Real

This section may be hard for some of you to read. You may be thinking that "getting real" doesn't apply to you, because you've been real about your weight issues for a long time now.

Sorry, but we *all* have blind spots.

At the same time, this section isn't about beating on you or criticizing you. Society has done enough of that, and if you're anything like the people who write to me seeking coaching, then chances are you've done enough of that to yourself over the years.

Getting real means getting beyond the usual insights most people have about themselves and about their weight. You have to take this to the next level. You are not overweight because you haven't found the right protein powder or fat burner pill, and this is true regardless of what you overhear at lunch with friends or at the office water cooler.

It goes without saying that the causes of obesity are myriad and complex. Pointing to any single external cause won't serve us. Does too much sugar, eaten consistently, contribute to fat gain? Yes, of course. That doesn't mean if we never ever have carbs again all our problems will be solved.

What we can say is that the sum total of our food choices has, up to this point, led us to where we are today.

Yes, maybe these choices go back to childhood, when you didn't know any better, and maybe you didn't have much of a choice. That is absolutely fair. But getting real means getting beyond the blame of your childhood and taking adult responsibility instead.

You need to stop playing the victim card and stop being the diet martyr. Life isn't fair. Get over it. Some people have better or worse genetics. Some people had more active lifestyles as children.

In terms of you losing weight, none of that really matters in the here and now.

While other people may be able to go out for dinner a few times per week and order what they want because they don't have a weight problem, that should not affect you or the choices you make. You are where you are.

Accept reality and accept responsibility for the journey ahead. Own the fact that when you choose a behaviour, you choose the consequences. Getting real is about getting past that point where you find it easier to complain about your weight or about the obstacles in your path than to simply ignore that mental noise and do something about it.

But keep in mind that thin, lean, and svelte people are not necessarily happy people, and they're especially not happy people because of their bodies. I have dealt with hundreds of lean people who look amazing, but who aren't healthy and whose lives are a *mess*. For many of them, their lives are a mess *because* of their obsession with their leanness and food and diets and all the rest.

Envy is not a wellness mindset, and the "grass is greener" mindset is always a lie.

This means we need to stop the compare, contrast, and compete game. That doesn't help you. It only hurts you. The people you might be envious of are often stuck in the very same compare, contrast, and compete game. Once you're stuck in it, the actual state of your body gets overlooked. It's never good enough.

Getting real means making all of this about you and *your* body, and what you are going to do about it moving forward. No one else needs to have a say.

As part of the get-real mindset, there's a quote you should write down and put somewhere you can see it every day. It's one of the best "get real" quotes ever written. Jim Rohn said, "If you really want to do something you will find a way. If you don't, you'll find an excuse."

Do a self-check now and again. Are you finding a way or finding an excuse? That is how you know if you are being authentic about how badly you want to lose weight.

Going Deeper

It's about getting beyond the surface of another attempt at weight loss via some random diet. Move past that.

For people who overeat, there is always what's called a primary or secondary gain in doing so. We don't just eat to satisfy physical hunger. If you overeat, ask yourself what the underlying reason really is. What's the *real* reason? It's more than just hunger and taste.

You have to be able to honestly look at what these payoffs are for you. I'll give you a hint: in my experience, these payoffs are almost always emotional in nature. There is a desire for some kind of emotional payoff. Food is acting as a kind of substitute. You just need to cut out food as the middleman.

We also have to get past the fact that this is all about willpower. Do you think you really have the energy to resist temptation and work to keep the weight off for the rest of your life? Doesn't that sound horrible? No one can do that! *No one.* Eventually, you should get to a point where you don't have to resist or struggle or even try. It should just be a habitual part of your lifestyle. Doesn't that sound easier?

At the same time, part of the get-real mindset is accepting that the journey to get to that place won't look exactly like you expect it to. There will be surprises. The path may not be the one you expect. The path may not be how you think it should be either. Getting real means accepting the path as it is, the one that is required of you— no more, no less.

At the bottom line, there are no big mysteries in all of this. Never buy into the "fast, easy, simple weight loss" gimmicks and books out there. You should be offended by such gimmicks! The insinuation that substantial weight loss can be fast, easy, or simple should be an *insult* to you because your own experience informs you that substantial weight loss is none of these things!

Aristotle said, "We are what we repeatedly do. Excellence, then, is not an act, but a habit." You have to develop healthy and self-nurturing habits and daily rituals that serve you and your goals. This is the only way to have substantial weight loss finally stop being something you have to try so hard at. It should become simple, as a result of lifestyle habits you have put in place.

Accept that there is never going to be a time when indulgent foods won't be appealing to you. Of course they will! They always will. But when you have a lifestyle and habits that serve you, you don't need to spend tonnes of mental energy "resisting" these foods.

We only get good at things we practice. Excellence may be a habit; but it needs to be practiced. Instead of spurts of perfection here and there, practice a healthy self-nurturing lifestyle every week. You may slip up here and there, and that's fine. This is not about being perfect. It's about sustainable, healthy choices that serve you and your goals. It's about being present and practicing things where you can learn from both your accomplishments and your slipups. There is no need for "perfection" in all of this. Let go of that kind of black-and-white thinking.

Carl Jung said, "Your vision will become clear only when you can look into your own heart. Who looks outside, dreams; who looks inside, awakes."

It's time to look inside and wake up. Looking at diets and their rules, or reading about good foods versus bad foods and supplements and all the rest—all of that is about looking outside. Look at how many diets and rules and debates there are out there. If that stuff worked, no one would struggle. These things can all be a *part* of your working solution, but they are not the whole of your working solution. That is what you have been missing until now. It's time to take a different approach.

Your Change Trigger

At some point there has to be an authentic "change trigger" deep inside you.

What this means is that you let go, and you accept that making this whole thing be about weight loss has never worked for you.

When you get real, you start to address all the deeper reasons you struggle with food, and all the deeper meanings that food has for you. But it all begins with some authentic "change trigger" where your soul tells you *we can't do this anymore*, and you finally listen to your soul's voice.

A great example of a change trigger is in the Hollywood movie *Rudy*. It is the true story of a diminutive underdog who dreamed of playing football at Notre Dame. No one in his blue-collar family took him seriously. But the death of his best friend was the "change trigger" for him to quickly pack his bags, move away, and go after his dream, even though he had no idea how he was going to do it or pay for it. On top of that, he lacked the grades to get into Notre Dame, and he lacked the size and the talent to be on the football team. Eventually he worked his way on to the team's practice squad and got to play in a game, living out his dream. In the process he earned a degree—the first person in his family to do so. It's a movie worth watching, or rewatching in the context of the power of a real-life change trigger.

Look beyond diets for your change trigger. Change triggers are something more monumental, and they are going to be deeply personal and unique to you.

For many people, their change trigger is hitting rock bottom. They get to a place where they are sick and tired of being sick and tired.

But it doesn't have to be anything that drastic.

I have had many change triggers in my life. One of my first ones occurred when I was deciding whether to go to university or not. When I was young I just didn't care one way or another because I wasn't mature enough to grasp the importance of such a choice for my future. During my first year at university, I was relatively aimless, with nothing really appealing to me as a course of study.

That summer, though, I got a job working in the same factory as my father. I hated it. I found it mind-numbingly boring, if not outright painful. I realized that if I didn't stay in school, then this kind of work was going to be my only option. That change trigger kept me in school; it helped me to find a major, and it set me on a career path.

One of my first mentoring students, Shara, was at one time a wannabe fitness and figure competitor. After several really terrible contest preps, she had suffered metabolic damage and was sick. It was a long way back for her. That experience was a change trigger for her to leave the bodybuilding and figure competition world entirely.

She ended up opening a personal training studio. It took off. Her studio got so popular, she had to expand to a much larger building. She now has several trainers that work under her. Her facility is extremely well known and well respected in her city, and she has developed a reputation as one of the only female trainers for athletes wanting to compete in MMA. Her athletes do very well, and she's even been interviewed on TV for the work she does.

Change triggers come in many shapes and forms. For example, it can be the end of a long-term relationship or even the loss of a job. I've had several clients whose spouses were alcoholics or otherwise substance dependent. These clients spent years trying to help their spouse get clean. Their marriage eventually dissolved in spite of the work they'd done to save it. But this served as the change trigger they needed in order to finally get real and lose the weight and keep it off. They were finally able to realize that they needed to be good to themselves, first and foremost.

Your own change trigger has to be something that resonates with you. It has to shake you up. A movie or a lecture or a big life-changing event could be a change trigger for you. As in the movie *Rudy*, the death of a friend or a loved one could be a change trigger. But only *you* can ever really know when you are experiencing a true change trigger in your life. It almost always leads to taking real action, the kind that you were never able to sustain before.

Chapter 2.
An Integrated Approach to Fitness

There's much more to fitness than the fact that physical exercise is good for your health.

Integrative fitness means being attuned to what your body and soul are telling you and then getting them both on the same page, and letting each support the other. When this happens, you'll experience noticeably better physical and mental health, as well as better peace of mind, and you'll find it easier to be more consistent with things like diet and exercise.

There's a giant difference between measuring your body and being authentically aware of (and in tune with) your body and soul. You can be "informed" about your body, about the number of calories you are eating, about how much you weigh, about your blood tests, about any medical conditions or physical ailments you have, but none of these things make you authentically "aware" of yourself.

Mindfulness or Mindful Awareness

Mindfulness or mindful awareness (in this book I use the terms interchangeably) is the outgrowth of integrative fitness. Mindfulness means establishing and practicing a **nonjudgmental** awareness of who you are, combined with an ability to listen to your body and mind.

This constant communication tells you how you are truly feeling and doing, inside and out. Your body is a source of tremendous wisdom. And isn't it true that you can benefit from any source of wisdom when you struggle with an issue? The wisdom of your body and soul is even more powerful for this particular issue, because it comes from inside you.

If you don't pay attention to these messages, who will? No one but you can be in tune with them. Your body is constantly talking to you. Your soul also talks to you—not just via your thoughts and emotions, but also through your physical body and your physical sensations. Listen, and learn to attune yourself to what they're saying, because both body and soul speak in gentle whispers.

If you ignore these messages, your body and soul *will* begin to shout at you, and sometimes scream at you. By that point, when you are practically forced to pay attention, you will already be suffering the consequences of ignoring them for so long. People get frustrated with their body whenever this happens, as if it were somehow working "against" them. That's not what's happening. Their body is trying to protect them and has been trying to do for a while now. They just haven't been paying attention!

I see this all the time in clients I deal with who have broken or damaged metabolisms. They hurt themselves by ignoring their own body's warning signs for too long. This is almost *always* a result of putting weight loss ahead of real health and well-being.

You can think of integrative fitness as a preventative measure. Someone taking a more integrated approach to fitness would never let that happen because they would be listening to their bodies and they wouldn't let it get that far.

According to integrative fitness, all of the physical systems of your body are in touch with the other faculties of your mind and emotions.

This is what I call the triangle of awareness. It

includes three realms:

- The mental realm
- The physical realm
- The emotional realm

These three realms of awareness are always working with and being affected by each other. Optimum health and optimum function result from the strength and the "fitness" of all three of these systems, both separately and together.

The more fit and conditioned each of these systems is, the better able they are to work together, as they should. The compound effect of this is amazing, so that the whole is much greater than the sum of its parts.

When you deplete any or all of these energy realms, it becomes harder for them to function optimally, and you get a negative feedback loop.

For instance, being substantially overweight is obviously going to be hard on your body, but the experience of this becomes hard on your mind and hard on your emotions. When normal daily tasks are more physically tiring for the simple reason that you're carrying extra weight around, it will also take more mental energy to do them. When it's the end of the day, and you're both physically tired and mentally tired, you suffer from loss of willpower, and small emotional struggles suddenly have much more of an effect on you.

This is part of what makes substantial and sustainable weight loss so challenging.

No fad diet will ever address this kind of thing, but it is a simple equation. Your mind is dependent on your body, and vice versa. You only have so much energy to go around. We often refer to this energy reserve as "vitality," but you can also think of it as the *experience* of vitality.

The more of this reserve you are able to regularly replenish, the better and healthier you are. On the flip side, the more you keep depleting this energy reserve, the more other aspects of your life suffer. The more various aspects of your life suffer, the more stressed you are, and the harder it becomes to replenish your daily energy and get back to experiencing real vitality.

The Goal of Integrative Fitness

The goal is to wake up every morning feeling that your body and soul are connected, instead of feeling like your body is somehow separate from you.

Mind, body, and spirit are intimately connected. The solution for substantial and sustainable weight loss lies in reconnecting these parts to the greater whole. The increased fitness of one element will support the greater fitness of the others. Don't focus only on the "weight loss," in other words.

Concentrating only on losing weight doesn't necessarily enhance your integrative fitness at all, and this is often where people come up short. A diet alone is too limited in scope to help you accomplish your goal of substantial and sustainable weight loss, for the simple reason that most diets ask you to ignore the mental and emotional realms, or to pretend they don't exist. But when that happens, eventually there's a rebound. There always is.

Dieting by itself, when considered in this larger context, solves nothing in the long term, even if you don't have any mental or emotional issues related to food or eating. When you combine a fad diet, and the subsequent rebound, with a preexisting mental or emotional issue related to food or weight (e.g. binge eating), it can make the negative feedback loop all the worse.

So you have to stop looking at diets themselves as solutions and start seeing the larger picture. This larger picture includes how and what you feel, and how and what you think.

A recent study [1] showed the importance of what's called "emotional ability" (what I've called emotional awareness) with respect to long-term weight loss. Those who had been trained in reading their own emotions did better than those who had only been given more nutritional knowledge. The researchers suggested that for people looking to lose weight, training in emotional ability was more beneficial than nutritional advice alone.

Diane Robinson, PhD, and Program Director of Integrative Medicine (!) at Orlando Health found that only one in ten dieters considered the emotional or mental health component of dieting when they began a diet. She said, "Most people focus almost entirely on the physical aspects of weight loss, like diet and exercise. But there is an emotional component to food that the vast majority of people simply overlook and it can quickly sabotage their efforts." [2]

This whole project is taking the above conclusions as its main premises: emotional ability or mindful awareness is the secret ingredient. Work on these things first. Consider the larger picture. And even when you do focus on a particular diet strategy (as we will do, later on), do it in a way that takes a more integrated approach.

Look at it this way: you wouldn't go for a week without feeding your body the energy it needs.

Well, you can't go for weeks on end without feeding your mind and spirit the energy that they need either. Hence the phrase, "Man does not live on bread alone." You need to use an integrated approach that "feeds" all three realms and keeps them all healthy and working together.

Here's the thing, though: this stuff has to start in the mind. I'll talk more about "how" to do this, but for now suffice it to say that you can consciously and purposely direct your thoughts, and this can reframe your attitudes and experiences. You need to use and directly employ language that is about silver linings and affirmative thinking, instead of thinking strategies that are all about grey skies or about worrying and focusing on your weight.

I've used it before, but a passage from the Bible comes to mind. Philippians 4:8 reads: "Finally, brothers and sisters, whatever is true, whatever is noble, whatever is right, whatever is pure, whatever is lovely, whatever is admirable—if anything is excellent or praiseworthy—think about such things."

(Later on, you will actually see how similar this Bible verse is to Buddha's eight steps to end suffering!)

For now, in terms of integrative fitness, I just want you to examine how your thoughts and feelings about your weight up to now reflect that Bible quote above. Has your thinking about your weight ever been about what is lovely, praiseworthy, right, or pure? Are these what you have focused on?

Can you see how negative or abusive thinking about weight loss takes you further and further away from the healthy perspective that can actually help you finally solve the issue?

You have to learn how to change your mind in order to change your body. You have to get yourself beyond "diet-mentality madness" and into an integrative fitness mindset. It all starts with relying on the messages your body and soul are delivering to you all day long.

Getting There

Learning to listen to your body means practicing being a good listener.

You have to stop and absorb and consider a message before you respond to it, and you have to practice doing this.

Think of it as the difference between stopping to think and read a serious email before writing a careful and considered reply versus being in a heated discussion where both parties aren't really hearing each other.

If you've attempted weight loss before with a fad diet, then up to now you've likely not been truly listening to your body, not in real terms. You've been trying to dictate to it. That's what most diets ask you to do.

Listening to your body means that you don't need to judge and attach baggage to these messages. Just start *considering* them. That's all!

Being aware means meeting yourself where you *are*, not obsessing over where you *want to be*. (As we shall see, one of the things Buddha emphasizes is that great want or great desire is the source of great suffering.) Listening to yourself from the inside out is the way to become your own best friend and to make sure you're in tune with your body's most important messages.

This doesn't mean you have to "like" every message your body and soul are trying to communicate to you. But you *do* have to start considering them and paying attention to them. Going through life "tuned-in" like this will deliver more peace of mind, and, frankly, more success.

The self-investigation section of this project will help facilitate this connection for you. But for now, to get this all going, you can try to actually *practice* some of what I've been talking about. Just stop, and listen. Meet your body and see where it's at. Consider it. Determine how you will respond and what that means for you going forward in any kind of diet strategy.

Your body and soul will appreciate it, and that will make weight loss much easier and more sustainable.

Note that this doesn't mean it is necessary to analyze, critique, or judge what you are noticing. Of course not! Instead, just notice what you notice. To go back to the email metaphor, don't overanalyze it, looking for hidden meanings, because frankly, your body doesn't speak with hidden meanings and passive-aggressive innuendo. People might do those things, but your body won't.

You also don't have to fully understand everything at first. Just listen. Try not to overthink it. If you have a thought or reaction, keep in mind you don't even have to believe every thought you have either. Ask yourself where a particular self-sabotaging thought came from.

Remember, communication is one part speaking and one part listening. Communicating with yourself and your body works exactly the same way.

Having a dialogue with yourself (that is, with

your *whole* self, including your mind and body) about your weight, or even having a dialogue directly with your weight, as if it were a person sitting right next to you, is another means of enhancing mindful awareness and bringing the root of your weight issues to the surface of your consciousness.

At first it's not even about finding solutions so much as it is just about getting the full issue out there in the open. The "true" solutions tend to reveal themselves after the issue has percolated for a while. That can take time. You just have to allow it.

Also, let's not forget that emotions are information as well. Emotions provide cues and clues about all the elements of your life: your body, your environment, your relationships, and your sense of self.

Emotions provide you with insight you can't find with rationality alone. You can learn to recognize, own, respect, understand, and even cherish your emotions as a means of profound self-connection.

Stop thinking that certain emotions can destroy you; emotions are there to serve you, not the other way around. Emotions are fantastic servants but tyrannical masters.

Even from a physical standpoint, your emotions are there to help you and provide you with insight. For example, if everything just seems more emotionally charged, it might mean you're drained in other ways. Feeling stressed and being drained of energy literally causes us to have more emotional reactions to all aspects of our lives. Even a movie can seem sadder than usual if you're physically and mentally drained.

In terms of emotional fitness and its connection to weight loss, remind yourself of this phrase: "If it's on your mind, then it's on your body; and if it's on your mind then it's *in* your body as well." What this means is that thinking and feeling are, quite literally, functions of your body. They are affected by the material wellness *of* your body, and they affect that wellness in turn.

You can calm your emotional centres by delving into them with calm energy. Emotional stresses, depression, and anxiety weaken your resolve. This means that being depressed or stressed about your weight can actually sabotage how consistent you will be in doing something about it.

If you have other unresolved emotional issues as well, then it is imperative to work through them, and to do so with calm energy.

The main cause of bad feelings, and the main intensifier of anxious feelings, is fear. Fear causes you to try to repress or avoid negative feelings, instead of facing them and dealing with them so that you can move forward. Fear is one of the most disabling emotions there is. The more you feed it, the larger and stronger it grows.

The way to deal with fear is to treat it for what it is: information. If you're experiencing fear, accept it, acknowledge it, and know that it can often signal something going on below the level of your conscious awareness.

The path to dealing with negative emotions is, oddly, *not* to focus on them. You do not struggle against them. You acknowledge them and accept them for what they are and for the insight they provide, and then you move on.

What you move on *to* are alternative thoughts and behaviours. You emphasize thoughts, feelings, and behaviours that serve you and your goals. This is self-directed thought and action. It is the topic of the next chapter.

Chapter References

[1] Kidwell, Blair, Jonathan Hasford, and David M Hardesty. "Emotional Ability Training and Mindful Eating." *Journal of Marketing Research* 52.1 (2015): 105–119. Web.

[2] Robinson, Diane. "Lose Weight by Focusing on Mental Health First." *Orlando Health*. N.p., n.d. Web. 17 Feb. 2016. <http://oh.multimedianewsroom.tv/story.php?id=1103&enter=>

Chapter 3.
The Self-Nurturing Mindset

What you will see emphasized again and again in this project is the concept of self-nurturing.

The self-nurturing mindset that will help you lose weight is a "get-real" mindset combined with self-supporting thoughts and emotions. This means you still have ownership of personal responsibility, but you use self-nurturing and self-supporting thoughts and emotions to hone that personal responsibility.

Up to now, when it comes to your weight, you have likely been in a self-rejecting, self-judging, and negative mindset. These things can never help you reach or sustain weight loss. That kind of energy will only beget more of that kind of energy.

For example, think about what happens if you

show a bit of kindness towards a stranger. Say you're in line at Starbucks. If you're kind and considerate, what kind of energy do you tend to get in return? Kindness and warmth tends to beget more kindness and warmth, doesn't it? On the other hand, if you are hostile and angry and frustrated with a stranger, well, what kind of energy does that tend to return you? Emotional walls come up. Nasty things get said. Everyone goes home angry.

Your interaction with your own body works exactly the same way.

Your body responds kindly and considerately to kindness and consideration. Remember that! Can you truly say you've treated your body with kindness and consideration in all your previous weight loss attempts? I'm willing to guess the answer to that is a resounding *no*.

Negatively judging yourself serves no purpose, except to keep you feeling inadequate and feeling like you're not good enough. Harshly judging yourself about your weight doesn't motivate you; it just depresses you. This is not the way to sustainable change. Stop the assault and battery inside your own head.

As I said before, this doesn't mean you have to like where you are. It just means that battering and abusing yourself for where you are at won't help. If anything, it will only contribute to the problem.

Think of a child acting out. You may not like what the child is doing, but the solution is *not* to verbally abuse him or her. (You can even find studies showing that verbal abuse doesn't help [3].) That would be horrific! Love and nurturing are often exactly what's needed, and exactly what's missing in such instances. Sure, there might be times where he or she is just testing boundaries, and what's needed is some firmness, but even then it should come from a place of nurturing and love, shouldn't it?

Responsibility is different from negative self-judgment and self-rejection. These things actually clutter and confuse real responsibility. They add tremendous emotional pressure. Get your mind right, and your body will follow.

As we talked about in the last chapter, simply paying attention to yourself and the messages your body is telling you is a form of self-nurturing. Of course, this is not the same as self-absorption in your own problems and issues. It won't serve us to feed into narcissism, or the idea of being a diet martyr, or things like that.

Self-nurturing is not about being selfish. It's about being self-ful. To be self-ful means being helpful and supportive to yourself and your needs. When you do that, you're better able to help and support the other people in your life.

Being self-ful means enriching yourself and appreciating yourself. This starts inside your own head. When you are very overweight, then a burger, fries, and a shake do not represent *real* self-nurturing; they are a substitute for it. Authentic self-nurturing comes from within. Food doesn't provide it.

Self-nurturing clears the way for greater clarity of thought. The more clarity you have about an issue you face, the better equipped you are to get to the root of the problem and deal with it appropriately. This is the mindful approach. Remind yourself that diet strategies are only part of all this.

When you have a true self-nurturing mindset, the goal has to stop being about specific numbers. The goal can no longer be about losing 40 lbs., 50 lbs. or 100 lbs. It can't be about reaching a certain bodyfat percentage. Numbers do not reflect a quality of life!

The goal has to be about living better and treating yourself better in your thoughts, feelings, and behaviours. You need to adapt to living a lifestyle that allows you to find out who you are and what you are about when you aren't worrying or obsessing about your weight.

Imagine what other and better things you could think about and that you could do if you weren't thinking about diets, dieting, willpower, food scales, and weight scales.

Things like scales are meant to be tools. They are no longer tools if you obsess about them, fear them, or you are tired of them, or exhausted by them. No carpenter sits at home at night obsessing over and fearing his screwdriver or his toolbox!

Imagine being able to replace all your concerns about diet and your weight with other, more invigorating thoughts.

How free would your mind be if you did just that? A free mind is a strong mind. A strong mind is a decisive mind. By contrast, a worried mind is a burdened mind. As the song says, free your mind and the rest will follow. Unlock any mental and emotional chains related to weight loss and stinkin' thinkin'. Break free and *be* free.

Your biggest ally in all of this is self-trust. That is your starting point. It can't start with calories, and grams, or percentages of bodyfat. Those are distractions, not solutions.

When you feel better about yourself, you don't need excuses or rationalizations. You stop hiding behind them. When this happens, you're free to gather serious spiritual momentum. Momentum is more powerful than willpower can ever be.

When someone has a slight hiccup in their diet, they feel negative because they think it means they "lack willpower." But this just isn't the case. If you keep thinking that when you cheat on a diet, it means you lack willpower, then you are forgetting about all the consecutive meals and days when you were consistent with your diet. You're judging yourself too harshly.

Willpower by itself is an easily exhaustible resource. Research proves it over and over again. This means that willpower can get you going on a project or a course of action, but it can't *keep* you going for very long. When and if other distractions come into your day, like work conflicts, relationship issues, and whatever else it may be, these things tap and exhaust willpower as well.

This is why self-nurturing is so important. It takes you away from a total and unrealistic reliance on willpower alone and the self-judgment that often accompanies it. So if there is a hiccup (and there will be, because no human being is perfect) you can learn from it and move on.

When you cheat on a diet even when you "don't want to," and you "know" you will feel bad about yourself for doing so, that tells us something. It tells us it's time to realize there is an emotional component to what's going on.

There is a *reason* that you are doing it. You need to look for what that reason is. Paying attention to your body and your emotions is how you do this.

In psychology this underlying reason is known as a "secondary gain." It means that when you cheat on your diet (for example), even though rationally you don't actually want to, there is some secondary payoff in it for you, *somewhere*.

Our job is to find it and deal with it.

That payoff is almost always meeting some kind of emotional need. Comfort, distraction, numbing, and avoidance are the common ones.

Of course these all represent a need for—you guessed it—self-nurturing.

Getting into a self-nurturing, self-accepting mindset means letting go of the perfectionist mindset, as well as the unrealistic idea that dieting is an all-or-nothing proposition. Let go of all the self-judgment that comes with diet indiscretions.

Accept that they will happen and learn from them. Try to learn why and how they happened, and what you can do better next time to prevent it. You can only examine a diet indiscretion in this way if you let go of the usual emotional self-recrimination and focus on true self-nurturing.

Willpower, Self-Nurturing, and Food Sneaking

Many people with a lot of weight to lose become "food sneakers."

I have had a lot of experiences with this with clients.

You sneak food because of some idea that other people are watching and judging you over your food choices.

Often, certain scenarios will trigger food sneaking. For instance, during the holidays, many clients will stress and worry over the food that will be present at parties and social gatherings. They stick to their diets and don't eat the indulgent foods at the parties, but the food they're not eating is all they can think about, so when they go home they binge in private. This is one of those examples where willpower is exhausted and spent in one area and leaves a person vulnerable later on. It's also an example of food sneaking. They didn't want to cheat in public, but in private it somehow seemed okay.

Most people who are food sneakers do it in private. They'll only grab a cookie when no one is looking, or binge in private when the family is away or asleep, that kind of thing.

I've actually had clients hide food in a closet and eat in the closet as well!

Being a food sneaker only intensifies the connection between shame, guilt, and the eating experience. It goes without saying that this isn't healthy. It's another example of having a thinking and feeling issue about food and diet.

If you are a food sneaker, it means there is some emotional "shaming" going on around food or eating. That mindset will never provide you a healthy way out of your struggle to lose weight. It's all a projection—you feel others are judging you when in truth you are judging yourself and projecting your judgment onto others.

If you feel uncomfortable or ashamed of eating in front of other people, that discomfort will be something you internalize. Every time you sneak food, your taste buds enjoy it, and it might have some emotional "secondary gain," but you shame yourself for it at the same time.

The clients I've had who were able to lose substantial weight were always the ones who were able to let go of any kind of negative self-judgment because of their weight.

You can assess yourself as being overweight

without having this fact damage your self-acceptance and self-respect. You can accept that you are overweight and that you no longer want to be. That is fine and understandable. But such an assessment must be free of negative self-judgment or negative emotions.

Athletes don't achieve greatness by constantly telling themselves, "I suck!" or "I'm terrible at this!" or "I hate myself." Achievers just don't think in those terms. Indeed, if they even approach that kind of thinking, it can put them in a long rut where they can't get their groove back.

Feeling good about yourself is always the better proposition for accomplishing something. The self-nurturing mindset is imperative for long-term success with this stuff. There is no way around that.

I'll conclude this section by emphasizing that adopting the self-nurturing mindset isn't like flipping a light switch. It *will* take time. That's what the self-investigation and questionnaire exercises are for.

At times, you'll find negative thoughts coming in. When that happens, those thoughts can be information. You can use them.

Chapter References

[3] Wang, Ming-Te, and Sarah Kenny. "Longitudinal Links Between Fathers' and Mothers' Harsh Verbal Discipline and Adolescents' Conduct Problems and Depressive Symptoms." *Child Development* 85.3 (2013): 908–923. Web.

Chapter 4.
Mindfulness and the Buddhist Approach to End Suffering

Now we get to the crux of the matter of solving substantial weight-loss issues.

If you have struggled with weight for years, it is *this section* that can free you from your struggle.

Let's be straight here. Even if you wanted to argue that what I am calling the North American diet mentality has worked for other people, if you are still struggling with weight, then it hasn't worked for you.

Stop seeing this struggle as a character flaw. It isn't. Our culture tells us it is, but it's lying. It's wrong. Instead, reframe your struggle and consider that maybe the approach that *might have* supposedly worked for others, some of the time, just doesn't work for you. It's the approach that is flawed.

The mindfulness approach is what you need. It's just a different way of perceiving your weight issue and what you're going to do about it. It's a different perspective on the issue itself, which in turn gives you a different approach to solving it.

We are thus going to use the Buddhist approach to end suffering as your personal approach to solving your substantial weight loss issue.

There are two different elements we need to address in order to get you to understand this shift in thinking. First, even though I've already talked about it, I want you to *really* understand the concept of mindfulness, or mindful awareness. After that, I want you to use the eight steps to end suffering as a long-term approach to solving your substantial weight loss issue.

Mindfulness

Jon Kabat-Zinn describes mindfulness as a lens. He writes that you can "think of mindfulness as a lens, taking the scattered and reactive energies of your mind and focusing them into a coherent source of energy for living, for problem solving, and for healing."

Think about that quote for a minute. That's what we want to do: take any scattered or "reactive" energy in our minds and *focus* them into a source of energy for problem solving and healing.

Mindfulness is about reflecting and thinking about our minds, our thoughts, our bodies, and our physical sensations. It's about using and thinking about our thoughts proactively, so that they don't use us.

Remember a diet can only be a part of the bigger picture. It isn't the whole picture. You need to let go of the idea that you have a food problem. You don't. You have a thinking and feeling problem *about* food, diets, and dieting. Mindfulness and mindful awareness is the way to solve this.

I know there is at least a part of you that would really rather just forget all this mindfulness stuff and just lose all this weight for good, thank you very much. But for now I need you to forget the wish list of what you "want" in the here and now, as well as what you wanted yesterday. These "wants" don't work for you. Instead, they torment you. (You'll see below that this is the Second Noble Truth.)

Let go the wish list. Move on to practicing the eight steps outlined below. Part of mindfulness is expecting mistakes. The difference is that with mindfulness training, you move beyond emotional self-judgment for these mistakes and instead employ your own rational mind to learn from them.

Furthermore, forget the wishbone proposition that you can live forever only eating foods that are "good for you." You aren't a food zombie, and learning to be more mindful won't turn you into one.

All these wishbone fantasies lead you to frantic and disconnected mental energy. Remember, we want to be able to focus our energy. Frantic mental energy leads to frantic actions and behaviours, and the end result of this is always (eventually) self-sabotaging behaviour. Aren't you tired of living in that cycle?

Instead, learn calm, patient energy. That is the path to mindfulness and awareness. Remind yourself that substantial weight loss is something you want to maintain for the rest of your life. So you need to adopt the kind of mental and emotional energy that nourishes this as a sustainable reality.

Calm, patient energy is at the heart of mindfulness. The wishbone mindset only creates "want," and this kind of want is a form of suffering because it leads to self-torment. You've likely lived it for years already.

The solution starts with reconnecting to yourself, because it is so easy to disconnect in our day and age. It takes awareness and mindfulness to reconnect and to stay connected. As with anything else, awareness takes discipline and it takes practice.

As I said earlier, the way to achieve deeper awareness is to "Sit, stay, and heal." This just means taking the time to calmly think about what you are thinking about and how you are thinking about it. You can't do that if you are always on the go inside your own head.

Wishbone thinking will keep you in a frantic energy space. Your backbone thinking will ground you.

Mindful awareness is about examining your thoughts. You will come to realize that you don't have to believe every thought that goes through your mind. Be aware of your thoughts, especially the ones that torment, bother, or sabotage you. Be aware of which thoughts are so unrealistic that they make you lie to yourself about what is possible.

Develop the habit of talking back to these kinds of thoughts, not with negative emotional energy, but with calm, rational alternative thoughts that serve you. This helps with mental fitness and with self-directed thinking.

What you will learn through mindful awareness is that when you make mindful choices that correspond to your own calm self-direction, the result is peace of mind. No diet can give you that. People often wrongfully *look* for it there, but that's because of the wishbone mindset.

Mindful choices come from within. This is what the eight steps to end suffering are all about.

Make no mistake here. Your attitude is a huge determinant in all things and all matters of your life. Your attitude is a mental state that predisposes you to think, react, and behave in certain ways. Embrace the adage, "Everything you do is infused with the attitude with which you do it."

The Buddhist Approach to End Suffering

People are often intrigued by a Buddhist or Zen approach. Other people reject it instantly as "airy fairy" new-age nonsense. I'd argue that there's nothing "new" about these philosophies, as they're thousands of years old.

All such an approach boils down to is taking a different philosophical approach than the one you have been taking for years—the one that hasn't worked, in other words.

The Buddhist or Zen philosophy gets you to focus specifically on what "is" instead of what you want or where you want to be. This approach gives you the proper tools for self-engagement in a process that includes personal growth while you solve an issue of struggling and suffering.

The North American approach assumes that life is a battle and you must fight to overcome all issues. According to this approach, life is all about winners and losers. That mindset and philosophy comes with tremendous emotional pressure.

The Buddhist mentality is about replacing the energy of resistance with the energy of acceptance. It means you don't have to like where you are at, but you accept it, and work with it.

You replace a battle mentality with the energy of "letting go" and "letting flow." The eight steps to end suffering are all about creating a flow of energy, kind of like a circle that keeps completing itself and gets stronger each time it does so.

Another benefit of the Buddhist approach is it gets you to stop compartmentalizing your weight issue as being only a weight issue. You come to accept it as a "you" issue, and that includes all the elements that make up "you."

When you work on "you" in positive and self-nurturing ways, you don't need to battle your weight. The battle mentality becomes irrelevant as you choose to just take care of yourself.

I have been using this Buddha approach to end suffering with my clients for years. I tend not to lay out the eight steps as we go along. When clients check in with me, I often challenge their thinking and reorient them on this path to end suffering.

When they got caught in the trap of want and desire, which gets them down on themselves, I remind them how useless that level of energy is for sustaining motivation and positive momentum. The path to end suffering is all about staying in the present and gaining momentum from the insights that the "process" provides.

When you only think of some far-off goal, you stray from being present and aware, and that is often precisely what ends up unraveling your resolve. If you think about your previous attempts at weight loss, you can likely identify all the times you went off track. It is almost always because you start focusing on the end goal rather than remaining truly present in task-oriented and process-focused consciousness that takes care of the now so that "later" takes care of itself.

This is also what the Buddhist philosophy to end suffering does. So let's examine it as it relates to weight loss.

The Four Noble Truths

First, there are four noble truths that underlie the eight steps to end suffering. The four noble truths break down like this:

First Noble Truth
Life contains suffering.
(This is sometimes better translated as "Life is stressful, or unsatisfying, or unreliable.")

Second Noble Truth
Suffering has a cause and the cause can be known.
(The desire and want for "more" is a common one.)

Third Noble Truth
Suffering can be brought to an end.

Fourth Noble Truth
The path to end suffering has eight parts.

Let's look at the path to end suffering in more detail. The path to end suffering is in eight parts because it will address eight aspects of yourself:

1) Your View, Perspective, and Perception

How do you look at your weight as a reflection of your lifestyle and the sum total of the choices you have made up to now?

2) Your Intention

What is the purpose you have behind ending the suffering of your weight issues? Is your intention based in self-rejecting, negative energy, or is it based in self-nurturing, self-directed energy?

3) Your Speech

This is not just what you say to others, but also the words you use to talk to *yourself*. When you think about your weight, is your internal language laden with emotional and judgmental words? Do you actively think about the language you use inside your own head and modify it so as to be more empowering and positive? Trust me: this matters.

4) Your Actions and Behaviours

These are more often the direct result of the thinking and feelings that precede them. See above.

5) Your Livelihood

Are you living in a way that supports your goals to lose weight with self-nurturing? Will your living and livelihood support you supporting yourself?

6) Your Effort

Are your efforts the result of positive, self-directed thought and intention, or the result of self-rejection, self-judgment, self-measurement, and unstable emotional wants and desires?

7) Your Mindfulness

Are you examining your thoughts with calm and patient energy, or are you letting them run wild? Are you thinking about what you are thinking about? Are you staying present? Are you staying aware? Are you practicing awareness? Are you infusing your self-directed thoughts with affirmative energy?

8) Your Concentration

What is your focus, and what kind of energy is influencing that focus? Is it flowing energy? Is it calm, patient energy? Or is it erratic, frenzied, anxious, and worried energy that taints and disrupts your focus?

When it is all laid out for you this way, can you see how addressing these eight elements of yourself can keep you present and self-directed towards solving weight issues?

The eight steps to end suffering are all about recognizing the importance of changing your mind to change your body. In Buddhist terms, we would call that right perspective and right intention. To get the body you aim for, you have to believe first in the importance of changing your mind.

The eight steps together create a circle that supports itself. Right mindfulness leads to right action and right livelihood and so on, and this all reinforces right mind all over again. Keep thinking of the eight steps to end suffering as a circle that keeps completing itself.

Let's examine the eight steps, then, with emphasis on how they relate to weight loss.

1) Right Perspective

Right perspective is about getting real about getting real.

If you want something different from your life than what you are getting right now, then you have to change your mental software—there's no way around this. How many diets do you have to fail at before you realize that a diet is not the "get-real" path? You have to update your thinking. Reprogram you mind with greater self-awareness, as well as greater awareness of your environment, your circumstances, your beliefs, and your intentions, and how all these things affect your ability to stay consistent on a reasonable diet strategy and lose weight.

You also have to accept that your "thinking" is a biological function. If you think better, you will act better. If you act better, you will feel better. If you feel better, you will think better—and then you keep reinforcing that positive feedback loop. You have to remind yourself that moods, emotions, and thoughts all affect the physical body and vice versa. And once you realize this, how does a focus *only* on your weight make sense? This is what Buddha meant by "right concentration" and "right intention" to end suffering. This is all part of right perspective and right view as well. Each step touches upon the others.

2) Right Intention

The Buddhist approach as I am describing it here is synonymous with a Zen approach or a Tao approach. What all of these have in common is getting rid of mental and emotional nonsense and clutter.

Mindfulness is about bringing more conscious awareness to every moment and to as much of your inner world as possible. This is how to live more fully, more completely, and more competently. This is "right intention." It is this expanded level of competence that will help you work the process of achieving substantial weight loss. No diet in the world can provide that to you. Every diet out there is just a description of a process. *You still have to work the process.* It is precisely this working of the process that gets results.

Right intention also means that you stop focusing on what you don't want and you focus instead on what you *do* want for yourself. This means self-directed thought, and it means focusing on supportive and self-nurturing thinking that always directs you towards what you do want, instead of thinking that is always trying to battle against what you don't want.

3) Right Speech

Right speech is what ties it all together. How you talk to other people and how you talk to yourself inside your own head when it comes to your weight is *everything*!

Right speech is what directs your thoughts and what energizes them. This is way more than just positive thinking. Right speech is so important that we are going to devote a big chunk of the next chapter to it when I cover Karl Albrecht's four habits to increase mental productivity and self-directed thought.

4) Right Actions and Behaviours

You should be able to see how the above three elements will positively influence you towards right action. Right actions and right behaviours must occur for the right reasons. This means you can't diet because you "hate being overweight." You can't diet because you "hate yourself for being fat." These would not be the right actions because they would be tainted by the wrong mindset.

Right behaviour means self-nurturing behaviour. At the same time, it doesn't mean self-indulgent behaviour. **Right behaviour,**

then, also means get-real behaviour.

Yes, this means structure and regimentation when it comes to diet. It also means consistency and compliance, and not just when you feel like it or when it's easy to do. Right action and right behaviour reflect right livelihood.

Right action and right behaviour are often about the details and logistics. If your struggle is with weight, then right action and right behaviour must include regularly established meal times. Right action and right behaviour must include regular and consistent sleep hygiene. Right action and right behaviour must include regular and consistent healthy, whole food meal choices, at the same time as it includes taking and finding the time to *prepare* those meals, sometimes in advance. This is right behaviour and right action, and it reflects right mindfulness. It marks the difference between self-indulgent behaviour and self-nurturing action.

5) Right Livelihood

Right livelihood reflects the sum total of all your right actions and right behaviours above. In short, if you want to "be" healthier and leaner then you must live the lifestyle of a healthy lean person. Right livelihood covers the details of all your behavioural choices added together, but it also covers livelihood on a much broader scale.

I had a client who worked irregular hours that often meant the graveyard shift. He complained about it for years, even as he got heavier and heavier and had sleep and other issues. He *talked* about how important these things were, yet he continued working a shift that prevented him from achieving his goals. Finally, he quit his job and found something else, even though at first it meant less pay. His health improved and he lost weight, and it wasn't long before his pay had increased as well.

You simply can't live like a person who doesn't care about their weight, and then turn around and claim that you *do* care about it. Your livelihood must support your health and well-being, or it's simply not the right livelihood for you.

Right livelihood isn't just about your workday or your career. Right livelihood is about having these things work and fit and be in balance with the live you live.

I find this is a very, very difficult thing for a lot of overweight people to accept. The get-real mindset is about accepting change on change's terms, and not as you think it should be. This is often lost on people who are not willing to choose "right livelihood" to end their suffering, because they unconsciously perceive the costs as being too great. But then, what are the costs of continuing to suffer?

Buddha makes no illusions that the path to end suffering can require serious sacrifice. He also notes that most people continue to suffer because they choose to not make the necessary sacrifices to end suffering. As Buddha put it, "Pain is inevitable, suffering is a choice."

On the other hand, I have had dozens of clients who fell in love with fitness. They thought the next logical step of this passion was to become personal trainers. But training others all day long left them no time to train themselves. And being in the gym all day sapped their energy for staying in that environment to train themselves; they couldn't wait to leave. They found that sometimes you can have too much of a good thing. But after they left personal training and found another career path, fitness went back to being something positive they did for themselves.

I am not saying everyone who is overweight needs to quit his or her job. I have clients who work shift work but have great bodies. I have clients who are on the road for two thirds of the year, but they stay near ripped year round.

What I am saying, though, is that you do need to address, *in real terms*, how your job or livelihood affects your weight. And you need to get real about what needs to change, whether it's the job or career, or just certain aspects of your job. (You can bet that my successful clients who have a lot of dinners out with *their* clients don't drink lots of alcohol just because everyone else is, for example.)

6) Right Effort

As I mentioned above, your efforts have to be infused with a positive and affirmative attitude. Your efforts also need to be about moving in the direction you want for yourself.

Your right efforts cannot be about trying to move away from what you don't want; they have to be about moving towards what you *do* want.

In other words, your efforts can't be driven about what you "can't" eat, and trying to resist what you shouldn't eat. Right effort is about effort that moves you forward and towards something positive. Ask questions like, "What can I eat that will help me with my goals?" or "What can I do right now that will help me with my goals?"

Right effort is never about trying to resist moving backwards, but always about moving forward in a positive and empowering sense.

Right efforts are more about considering the bigger picture, and less about focusing on the struggle itself. Right efforts are never something you feel forced to do. Right effort is about knowing and embracing that your mind is involved in everything you "do," not just everything you think.

Right efforts also involve *how* you do these things. Right efforts are always quality efforts, but only when they are influenced by right attitude. (I'll return to this when I discuss right concentration.)

7) Right Mindfulness

Right mindfulness could be thought of as the state of mind of all the above elements coming together, such that the whole is greater than the sum of its parts. When all these elements of right mind and right direction are in sync, right mindfulness is the result.

In the state of right mindfulness you don't feel anxiety, worry, or chaos about your weight. Right mindfulness is self-direction on steroids. When you practice right mindfulness, and when you know and consistently experience the state of right mindfulness, eventually that becomes a state of being as well. At that point, your struggle and your suffering about weight become insignificant. The "struggle" is gone. It's a non-issue. You are simply moving towards something else, rather than still fighting against and resisting weight, food, cravings, or whatever.

But let me give you a very glaring celebrity example of the lack of right mindfulness. Oprah Winfrey is well known for cultivating the inner realm of spirituality and a can-do attitude. She was the first to extol the virtues of writers like Eckert Tolle. Her life story is also incredibly remarkable, in terms of what she's achieved and what she's overcome to do so.

Yet Oprah is also known for her struggle with weight.

A few years back, Oprah's magazine ran a cover story of Oprah with the caption, "How did I let this happen again?" and it was all about her gaining all her weight back… again. I read the article with interest, as I had been following Oprah's struggle with weight for years as an example of what not to do.

Here is what I mean. For years I have paid careful attention to what she says about her struggle with weight. I've read articles where she writes about her weight, and I have seen many of her interviews where she talks about it. There is one consistent theme that runs through all of them. She repeats *over and over* again how much she *hates* exercise. Yet as someone who is normally all about awareness, she has never connected that to her issue.

Think about it: How long can you engage with something you claim to hate? What level of attitude are you going to consistently bring to something that you claim you hate? Oprah exercises to control weight, even though she hates it. One time she trained for a marathon, but only as a goal to accomplish, not as something to simply experience.

That's a mindset of struggle. That mindset has kept her trapped for decades. I would be willing to bet that when it comes to the remarkable things she has accomplished in life, she has a different mindset entirely. I doubt she ever talked about how much she hated being on television or how much she hated the tasks involved in putting on a television show and building a media empire.

Can you see the difference in terms of right view, right perspective, right efforts, and right mindfulness, in regards to her struggle? Instead of hating exercise, what difference would it make if she partnered and connected with exercise, and experienced it as something deeper, something that was more than just something she "had" to do to control her weight?

On the flip side of right mindfulness and the self-connecting nature of exercise, a lot has also been written about mindful eating. I won't go too far into the concept here. Whole books have been written about mindful eating.

Mindful eating is all about eating with awareness and without distraction. It's about chewing your food more consciously. It's about putting your fork down between bites. It's about appreciating food and meal times. It's about knowing that "the banquet is in the first bite," as the saying goes.

The part about mindful eating that I want to talk about, however, is about your mindfulness *between* meals, and when it is *not* mealtime. Mindfulness in regards to food, diet, and weight loss is also about having better and other things to think about than food, calories, and diets.

If you establish regular meal times and prepare several of your meals in advance each day, then between meals there should be other and better things to exercise your mind with and to engage your mind over.

In terms of right mindfulness, I will conclude by saying that exercising and eating right aren't supposed to be things you obsess over or feel anxious about. They're supposed to be what you do to *relieve* stress and anxiety! That should be your goal with it. That is representative of right mindfulness and right intention.

8) Right Concentration

Right concentration is all about self-directed thought. This means focusing on thoughts, feelings, and behaviours that move you towards self-nurturing and towards your engagement in the process. That is right concentration.

Wrong concentration is focusing on resisting temptation, avoiding bad foods, trying not to think about hunger. If you focus on what you don't want, you only create more of that very thing.

There is an old Zen or Buddhist expression that says, "The universe responds in the affirmative," and "Your mind responds in the affirmative." What this means is that self-directed thoughts such as "Why can't I do this?" or "Why do I keep failing at weight loss?" or "Why am I so overweight?" will just have you seeking answers to those questions.

The answers to those questions won't move you towards the process of establishing substantial and sustainable weight loss! Right concentration is focusing on things like "How can I improve my commitment to my weight loss goal?" and "How is my dieting attitude going to be different this time?" and "What can I do better today to stick to my goals?"

If what you focus on expands, then this type of right concentration keeps you moving in the direction of a solution, instead of continuing to concentrate at the level of the problem. Your concentration level must be focused on affirmatives that move you towards investing and positively engaging in the process of weight loss. Focusing on how unhappy you are with your weight or on trying to resist indulgent foods are wrong concentrations that keep you focused at the level of the problem.

* * *

At some point, right mindfulness always leads to right behaviour and action, and you stop doing what you know doesn't serve you, doesn't help you reach a goal, and doesn't make you feel good about yourself. You start knowing the difference between useless self-indulgent behaviours that don't help you, versus positive self-nurturing choices that will serve you in the long term.

Now does all this happen in one fell swoop?

Of course not.

But it *can* start happening *today*.

The key word in developing any new ability is practice. Practice reinforcing your decision to "choose yourself" better and stop trying to "punish yourself" better. Then, just remind yourself to practice the behaviours that reflect this new and improved mindset. This is a great way to set limits that feel natural instead of forced.

Right mindfulness leading to right action is a process, not a goal. It takes time. Anything that takes time requires patience. Be patient with yourself. Go as slow as you need to go.

You aren't on *The Biggest Loser* competing against anyone else. Stop with the twelve-week total transformation madness.

Remind yourself that obsession is an absence of mindfulness. You can obsess about weight, or about food, or about your body, or even about all three at once. But this is not the same as being in control. It's not the real control and empowerment that mindfulness and the eight steps above provide.

Mindfulness means you control the whole scenario. Obsession means the whole scenario controls you.

As you practice the right mindset and the eight steps, you will realize that the less you think about weight loss as a goal to accomplish, the more you will see weight loss as a by-product of something much deeper and much healthier. (This is a reflection of "right intention.")

The less concerned you are with numbers and bodyweight changes, the more in touch you can be with a healthier thought process, and the more in touch you can be with the feelings and thoughts that help you (instead of always trying to move away from the feelings that hurt you). A focus on weight loss is no substitute for getting real about all elements of your life and seeing all of it as connected. That is what the journey from right mindfulness to right intention to right livelihood is all about.

It's the process that provides the insight, and it's this insight that you need to self-adjust and stay true to the process. The process provides insight into your body, insight into what tolerable hunger really is, what good energy is, and so much more.

The process is the goal and the goal is the process. Weight loss isn't just a goal, but the result of choosing to live, think, and feel differently than you have been.

When you get to this point, your mind and your body appreciate how good it is to not be obsessed by foods, by diets, and by weight scales and all the rest of it.

Yes, it *can* feel like hard work at first. Every worthwhile process usually does, and change never happens without hard work.

But this is a different kind of hard work. It's hard work that connects you with yourself, physically, mentally, and emotionally. Instead of being exhausting—as most diets are—it becomes *invigorating* hard work. It becomes hard work you do on behalf of nurturing yourself, supporting yourself, believing in yourself, investing in yourself, and doing better for yourself.

Chapter 5.

Karl Albrecht's Four Mental Habits to Increase Productivity

Raise your hand if you've lost some weight before now.

Yes, I imagine many of you reading this have lost weight at least once, before gaining it all back again. This *proves* that you have the fortitude to follow a diet for a given time period. Obviously, though, that's not all there is to it.

There is absolutely no doubt that mental habits, constructs, and patterns are hugely powerful, for either good or ill.

I should mention here that the self-investigation section of this project will go a long way to helping you create better, more productive, and healthier mental constructs.

Our goal is to make the transition from "weight-loss tourist" to "permanent resident." The only way to get there is to address your mental habits, structures, and patterns.

In Karl Albrecht's *Practical Intelligence* (2007), Albrecht outlines four key mental habits that can help you develop more effective mental productivity and self-directed thought and action. The four mental habits are a great addition or extension to the eight steps outlined in the previous chapter.

Practicing the eight steps, and practicing these four mental habits, combined together with the self-investigation and questionnaire section, can help you nurture powerful, productive, and useful mental habits that will help you lose weight permanently.

The Four Mental Habits

1) Mental Flexibility

This term means just what it says. As you can imagine, mental flexibility must by definition also include the *absence* of mental rigidity or stubbornness. Many people hold on to ideas for their need to "be right." As Aristotle said, "It is the mark of an educated mind to be able to entertain a thought without accepting it."

Mental flexibility is about freeing yourself from narrow-mindedness, dogmatic thinking, and judgments. It's about ridding yourself of fear-based avoidance of new ideas and experiences—say, the idea that it's not the "diet" that's the issue, or the idea that maybe carbs, proteins, and fats are *all* important parts of a balanced diet.

As Albrecht put it, "Mental flexibility is at the very foundation of your ability to perceive clearly, think clearly, problem solve, learn and grow as a person."

It's actually the rigid, fixed mind that is the most cluttered one. When you go from diet to diet trying to lose weight, you are exercising a fixed and rigid mind, not a mentally flexible one. A rigid mindset will think of foods in terms of good versus evil, allowed versus outlawed foods, and other mental constructs that don't serve you in your goal to lose substantial weight. A rigid mind might swap out one food for another, in terms of what gets vilified, but the thinking process is ultimately the same as it has always been.

A flexible mind will be better able to appreciate the integrative fitness approach. It will be better able to see that you can't simply compartmentalize "diet and fitness" as entities totally separate from the rest of your life, your lifestyle, and your mental habits. A flexible mind will be able to see fitness in new ways and rise above old patterns of thinking.

2) Affirmative Thinking

This one is key to moving you forward in terms of permanent and sustainable substantial weight loss. Affirmative thinking is about developing the habit of perceiving, thinking, speaking, and behaving in ways that support a healthy emotional state inside your own head.

Relative to what we looked at last chapter, you can think of affirmative thinking as being all about establishing "right mindfulness" and the self-nurturing mindset.

Daniel Amen said most people don't give their thoughts a second thought. Well, if you are overweight, you can't afford *not* to! If you are overweight, then how and what you think about food and your weight needs to change.

You want to not just examine your thoughts but also self-direct them towards affirmative thinking. Affirmative thinking also gets you into the practice and habit of directing your emotions as well. When you practice directing your emotions with affirmative thinking, this prevents your sabotaging emotions from directing you instead.

Affirmative thinking means being conscious of what you allow into your mind. By doing so, you develop a filter through which you can empower yourself and thus not be subject to circumstances or individual misperceptions that can sabotage you. This includes what people and places you allow to influence you.

For instance, your environment can be supportive, it can be neutral, it can be sabotaging, or it can be toxic to your goals. If this is the case, you have to recognize that. As with Buddha's "right livelihood," you may have to do something about it as well.

Affirmative thinking goes beyond positive thinking to something more concrete and deliberate. Affirmative thinking is about paying attention to your thoughts and knowing you don't have to believe every thought you have. I remind you again of that quote from Aristotle: "It is the mark of an educated mind to be able to entertain a thought *without accepting it*."

You don't have to accept it! Just entertain it, look at it, see it for what it is, and file it away for use later on. Or, if you don't think it serves you, by all means simply dismiss it.

This means paying attention to your thoughts and looking for thoughts and actions that serve you and thoughts and action that hurt you. For example, if you notice that surfing other people's Facebook pages makes you feel bad about yourself, this means that the behaviour is not "right behaviour" because it leads to thoughts that weaken and hurt you. If that is the case, you can simply choose to stop surfing other people's pages.

As another example, if looking at magazine pictures of perfect bodies makes you feel bad about yourself, then realize that this behaviour is not right behaviour because it leads to thoughts that disempower and weaken you. (Affirmative thinking would also acknowledge that comparing yourself to models who have dieted down to unmaintainable levels, used diuretics and other peaking strategies to lean out further, and then have been Photoshopped is not reasonable or realistic.)

Affirmative thinking involves two primary patterns of mental activity: selective attention and selective thinking.

Selective attention involves actively "censoring" what you allow into your mind and proactively choosing what you direct your attention to. This goes back to the Buddhist idea of "right concentration" or "right focus," and the idea that what you focus on expands. What are you paying attention to? What are you actively looking for? What environments are you immersing yourself in?

Selective thinking involves dwelling intently on the kinds of ideas, reasoning processes, conclusions, and intentions that are more likely to bring you positive results in your life.

Affirmative thinking is about looking at what thoughts and ideas serve you. Generally, this means focusing on positive, uplifting energy, because as we talked about earlier, like begets like. Toxic thoughts will beget more toxic thoughts.

However, at the same time, affirmative thinking is not just positive thinking. There's more to it. As I said earlier, affirmative thinking maintains a get-real mindset. The problem with positive thinking is that it isn't always thinking in real terms and about your actual reality. Not everything in life is positive or easy, but there are affirmative, self-empowering ways to frame and think about negative or difficult things.

This means accepting the reality of your current behaviour and your current actions. For instance, you might say to yourself, "I would like to take some horseback riding lessons," or "I would like to diet a little harder." But if you don't actually *do* either of those things, then those thoughts to yourself are untrue. When someone repeatedly lies to you, it's hard to trust them. The same is true if you lie to yourself.

What you need to remind yourself of is that outside of your work and personal responsibilities, what you are doing right now is what you really and truly want to do. You can't be sitting on the couch eating Doritos and telling yourself that you desperately want to diet harder, because your actions show that this is just not true. This is not affirmative thinking.

This is another reason to examine your own thoughts and realize you can't necessarily believe them. The reality of your behaviour must be taken into account. That is the first line of acceptance. Entertain thoughts, but when you do so, see them for what they are. Many might seem empowering, but upon closer inspection, are merely instances of want and desire. If so, reframe them to be more accurate or throw them out entirely.

If there is something you are doing right now that is not serving you well, like stopping at a drive-thru on the way home from work each evening, or if there is something you are *not* doing regularly that would serve you well, like getting up earlier so you can exercise before work, then you either need to change that behaviour, or you need to adjust your thinking and accept such behaviour for what it reveals about you.

Aristotle also said, "We are what we repeatedly do." For achieving and sustaining substantial weight loss, everything associated with that process must become habit.

Mental habits of affirmative thinking, selective attention, and selective thinking are what led to right action, right behaviours, right concentration, right intentions, and right efforts—all of which will go much further towards real-world weight loss than whatever's being shilled by the latest late-night infomercial.

3) Semantic Sanity

This is the habit of using language more consciously and deliberately, especially inside your own head. This relates to Buddha's "right speech." Practicing semantic sanity eventually leads you to stop torturing yourself with lies or negative emotions.

Semantic sanity is about thinking more clearly by searching for the right words, rather than reacting with whatever words pop into your head. Semantic sanity thus relies on calm, patient energy. It means stopping, pausing, and thinking about your thoughts and word choices *before* you react to them.

Revising the way you talk, especially inside your own head, helps you to revise the way you think. For instance, if you are someone who tends to opt for emotionally impactful words, then you might focus on framing things in more rational terms.

All of this feeds into Buddha's eight steps to end suffering. When overweight clients first come to me, most of them use phrases like, "I'm such a loser," "I feel like such a failure," "Why can't I do this?" and "I'm so lazy but I don't want to be."

All of these negative thoughts sap your self-esteem and demotivate you. They also give you a default position in your mind that you can't do it. At the first hiccup or obstacle, that will be the thought you turn back to first.

Let me put this more strongly: if you are such a failure, and such a loser, or you are so lazy… then why bother with *any* of this? You have pretty much already set up your mind to give in and quit. Just give up now!

Or, here's a better idea: get your head out of

your ass and *let go* this kind of stinkin' thinkin'! **This is priority number one.**

I use such strong—even vulgar—words above as an example of semantic power. How you talk inside your own head is *everything* when you have a goal. (You might be polite and positive when talking to other people, but how do you talk inside your own head?)

I've had many clients write me over the years, "I feel like such a failure." This is a pretty impactful choice of words, especially inside one's own head. I usually ask them to look at other areas of their lives and then tell me in light of what they find whether they still feel they are truly "failures."

Then I ask them to examine how that statement makes them feel. Does it motivate them? Does it inspire them? Almost always they say that the feeling weakens and paralyzes them.

Good. This means we're getting somewhere. We've already turned a potentially sabotaging thought into an insight.

I ask them to rephrase the statement "I feel like such a failure!" into something that is more accurate semantically and also more affirmative. Very often I have to help clients with this at first because their default mental habits are so ingrained.

So, "I feel like such a failure!" becomes, "I often slip up when it comes to my diet, though I am actually on top of so many other things in my life."

You can see how this is something we can build on.

It then leads to something like, "If I want to feel better and do better, then I have to think better and more clearly when it comes to my diet. I slipped up this time because *[insert reason]*, but then I let it continue by calling myself a loser, which only made me feel worse and sapped my motivation. It didn't serve me at all. What would a winner think?"

So, to take things further, we actually ask, what *would* a winner think?

"I've been consistent with my diet before. I have to think in terms of consistency now, too. From now on, I will tell myself *[insert something true and unique and empowering that reminds me to be consistent and do what needs to be done]*."

This is combination of semantic sanity and affirmative thinking is what you need. Notice how the improved thought process is less laden with negative emotional imprinting and self-judgment. It's realistic, so it doesn't shy from past mistakes, but it is still very affirmative. The thoughts are clearer and not as emotionally heavy, but they are still true.

Some people need extreme overhauls in their thinking when it comes to semantic sanity and affirmative thinking. Others only need some regular and consistent tweaking here and there.

For example, clients often report asking themselves something like, "Why can't I do this?" For many of my clients, that statement just needs to be tweaked a bit.

The statement, "Why can't I do this?" can become, "What do I need to address in order to be able to do this?" Or you can be more specific, "What can I address, right now, to be able to do this?"

This is self-directed thinking that is positive and affirmative and takes the person in a direction towards useful and insightful answers, and away from the focus on the problems and the mistakes.

As another example, I get clients who will write and say, "I was doing great on my diet, and then I had a cookie, and that led to finishing the whole box. I'm miserable because I've completely blown my diet and all my progress." Once again, a lot of this isn't even true, and it's laden with emotion that keeps those lies in place and makes the lies seem true.

First of all, there is no such thing as perfection with respect to a diet. So judging yourself as a failure if you don't diet "perfectly" is already a lie, and a damaging one. At some point, every person will indulge in foods that are not technically serving their interests when it comes to weight loss or keeping the weight off. That doesn't make you a failure; it makes you human! You need to account for this.

Next, when you unpack the above series of thoughts, you need to pay more attention to that initial affirmative thought: "I was doing great on my diet." For most of you in that above example, that first affirmative thought gets lost in the self-judging and negative thoughts that follow it.

That initial affirmative thought proves that you aren't a failure, and that you were making progress with consistency and commitment. That's powerful. Focus on that. (What you focus on expands, remember?)

The rest of the thoughts that follow that first affirmative thought don't disprove the initial one. That momentary slipup doesn't cancel the consistency that led up to it. In fact, missteps, hiccups, mistakes, stumbles—these are all part of the learning process in getting to "right livelihood" and "right mindfulness."

A slipup is just an indicator that "right actions" were not taken. That is something to investigate. Any high achiever will tell you they learn from their mistakes *more* than their successes. We always focus on the wins, but it's the mistakes where you learn. This is true in sports and for entrepreneurs and everywhere else you look, and it's true for dieting. Let go of the unnecessary emotions that come with mistakes so that you can learn from them and build off them.

You can do this by simply taking a moment to "unpack" your thoughts, then reframe them and redirect them towards something useful. It all starts with having enough awareness to "pay attention" not just to the sabotaging behaviour but also to the thoughts that led up to it and to the thoughts that followed it.

4) Valuing Ideas

This fourth mental habit of Albrecht's is a little more general, though it's obviously closely related to the previous ones, like mental flexibility. (Though hopefully you'll see how it's different by the end of this section.)

It's about seeing the potential in new ideas, instead of mentally and emotionally seeking reasons not to. It's about being able to challenge your own worldview at any given time. It means being strong enough to at least "consider" new ideas, even if they challenge your current belief system.

It goes without saying that if you have tried "every diet under the sun," and they haven't worked, then something about how you think about diets and dieting has to change. (That's why I place so much emphasis on a general diet strategy instead of this or that individual diet.)

When you value ideas, you see nuance and opportunity in everything. Valuing ideas helps you conjure new possibilities, where before you might have thought in terms of limitation. For example, consider my claim that you don't have a food, weight, or diet issue, but that you have a thinking and feeling issue *about* food, weight, and diet. Think about this and consider the *options* and *opportunities* within that idea.

I also want to emphasize the importance of not retreating into old patterns of thought. Restricted foods are not the answer for achieving and sustaining substantial weight loss. Instead, see the value and opportunity in taking the grander lifestyle approach to weight loss. Consider (or brainstorm) the options you have when you take a mindfulness approach.

In my opinion, valuing ideas is often about looking at the larger picture. Going to the bookstore and looking only in the diet and weight loss section is NOT an example of valuing ideas. It's an example of the "same mindset, different day" approach. Going from gluten-free to Paleo to "whatever else is in fashion" diet is not truly valuing ideas so much as looking for ways to stay within a comfort zone.

Many people claim to be willing to try a totally new approach, but what they really mean is they'll try a new approach only as long as it fits within their existing belief system. Many people email me telling me they're willing to "try anything," only to then list out twenty or more restrictions that this so-called "anything" must include!

Sometimes it doesn't come out until I send them their diet, and they say, "Oh, I can't eat this much food. I need a diet with less food to lose weight." Or they say something like, "My experience has taught me that I don't do well on more than 40 grams of carbs, max. I'll need something with less carbs."

These things are not actually true, but the client has been absolutely, positively convinced that they are true—partly from relentless marketing messages, and partly from simply misreading biofeedback and their body's own signals.

As another example, I will get clients who read my books and articles in advance and then join with my one-on-one coaching because they liked what they read and my different approach. Things get going, and they actually do pretty well for a time, but at some point many of them revert back to their previous diet mentality. They will write and say things like "I know the scale doesn't matter, but I haven't lost any weight in three weeks. I'm thinking of doing a nine-day cleanse… it's just to get the pounds coming off again. What do you think?"

My reaction is, "NO!" Trust the process! See the value—the opportunities and options—in simply letting your body acclimate to the new diet. There *are* things going on that you can't see, and which won't show up on the scale. Letting these things happen will bring positive results.

Here is another example: "Coach, my weight is still not moving. My vacation is only four weeks away at this point! What do you think about cutting carbs just for the next few weeks to get the weight loss going again?"

Again: No!

Trust the process.

It's easy to value different ideas "at first," but

it's much harder to act consistently on a new approach and to trust in the process without reverting to old habits. This often marks the difference between someone who is coachable and someone who isn't. A client can have much more weight to lose, or be starting with much more stacked against them, but if that client is truly willing to value ideas and new ways of thinking, they'll end up far better off than the client who is really just seeking validation for current ways of thinking.

* * *

When you can consciously observe and manage your own thinking process, you can arrive at better decisions, give yourself better options, and take more purposeful action. You'll find that you get fewer interruptions to your progress from unthinking impulses that have steered you wrong.

This is what Buddha means by "right mindfulness."

If you are trying to achieve substantial and sustainable weight loss, then you should be monitoring your thoughts and thought choices with as much or even more attention than you monitor your food and your food choices! Albrecht deliberately labels these four mental constructs as "habits," and that is what they need to become.

Chapter 6.
The Diet Strategy Mindset

I want to emphasize that embracing integrative fitness and the self-nurturing mindset must come first, before you really dig into any kind of diet strategy. And even then, a true diet strategy (as opposed to this or that fad diet) will embrace and enhance these things.

It is not that you have the self-nurturing mindset and "then" you have the diet strategy, as though these things were two, completely separate entities. Rather, the two go together.

To begin, here is what I want to focus on, with respect to your diet:

Learn to bring meal-by-meal mindful awareness to what you eat, why you eat, when you eat, and how you eat.

Write that last sentence down and keep it somewhere that you can see it (e.g., your fridge).

The truth is most of you who struggle with weight have been told to only focus on "what" you eat. Usually this is framed in terms of good foods versus bad foods, allowed foods versus demonized foods. This isn't healthy or realistic.

Suffice it to say that most people who have a lot of weight to lose have a complicated relationship with food. Maybe you fear or hate food, but you also love it. You want it and need it, but in the middle of a diet, you don't like admitting that, or are not sure how to deal with it. You probably also have many dual or contradictory thoughts about food, diets, and weight loss. These have to be addressed.

Food can and should be used to nourish the body, but food can be used to nourish the soul as well. Why do so many diet gurus refuse to admit this?

I do want to be careful. Context and mindset are everything, here. The same behaviour can mean different things, depending on the mindset behind it.

Having a Big Mac or a Whopper with cheese and fries and a shake on your way home from work or having several slices of leftover chocolate cake or a box of snack bars when you're feeling lonely at night isn't nourishing your body or your soul. These are attempts to satisfy emotional voids.

When these mindset issues are addressed in a real way, then these same indulgent foods (yes, including burgers or cake or ice cream) *can* be enjoyed from time to time, and they *can* provide real comfort and enjoyment, instead of being used as a self-medicating substance to mitigate emotions.

One person eats a few cookies, enjoys them, and moves on. The other eats one cookie, torments themselves over the "cheat," then has the whole box and feels even more miserable afterwards.

There is a huge difference!

Once you get to the point where food isn't used for satisfying emotional voids, then eating a large amount of these foods will no longer appeal to you as an emotional crutch. They certainly won't appeal to your body, either. By then food won't have a hold on you in terms of emotional torment or self-sabotage.

Eating should be about appreciation and enjoyment, as well as about calm self-connected energy. It should have nothing to do with negative emotions like fear, anxiety, worry, shame, and guilt. No other mammal on the planet has these negative emotions connected with their eating experience. That's a construct of our culture.

Accept and embrace that food is many, many things.

<blockquote>
Food is essential.

Food is survival.

Food is fuel.

Food is social.

Food is enticing.

Food is sensual.

Food is provocative.

Food is visceral.

Food is celebratory.
</blockquote>

Most important, food is abundant. It's everywhere.

You can't pretend that you are going to

become a diet zombie or that food is just fuel and nothing else. That's *nonsense.*

If that were true we wouldn't have issues with food at all, would we? This is about getting real. Food is all these things and more.

What you eat, *how* you eat, and *why* you eat are intertwined with issues about body image, control, self-control, your emotions, your family history, sensual pleasure, and all kinds of other unconscious realities that you need to make conscious and think about.

Food, and meals in particular, should be a pleasant experience free of guilt, anxiety, shame, mindlessness, torment, or fear. I may sound like a broken record, but I keep reinforcing this because it is that important. If you've tried dieting before, then what I'm talking about right now has likely been the missing link in all your failed attempts at substantial weight loss.

A Diet Versus a Diet Strategy

All these "diets" have focused on food, food, food, and nutritional advice. None of them focus on the real challenge: enhancing your emotional awareness and developing an empowered, useful, and healthy mindset towards food and eating. Following another diet without this is like trying to bake a cake without flour. This is why diets alone won't cut it for you.

This is why I talk about the difference between a diet and a diet strategy. A diet focuses only on food, on what's allowed and what's not. A diet strategy thinks about how we approach food and meals, food preparation, satiety, and so on. It goes hand in hand with your mindset towards eating.

Here are a few general guidelines.

First, eat at regular meal times. (And I mean "meal" times, not snack times.) Try to establish these and stick to them. It just makes sense biologically and mentally in terms of hunger to establish your own habits and routines.

On a related note, *have breakfast*. Breakfast remains the most important meal of the day. Remember the example of "Greg" at the beginning of this project. Greg skipped breakfast for most of his life, yet he never saw it as connected to his weight problem.

Eating breakfast gives you energy for the day, it affects your hunger and energy levels, and it gets all sorts of complicated systems inside your body working nicely. It also helps your motivation by starting your day off with eating a meal that's part of your overall diet strategy. It gets positive momentum going early.

Moreover, have some protein *and* some carbs at breakfast. A recent study looked at the benefits of having carbs at breakfast.[4] They compared a high-carb breakfast to a low-carb one. At first, the two groups showed similar amounts of weight loss. But after about week sixteen, the low-carb group started gaining back their weight, while the high-carb group continued to lose more weight.

The researchers also measured the ghrelin levels of the participants and found that the high-carb group had theirs drastically lowered. To make a long story short, lowered ghrelin makes you less hungry and makes you experience fewer cravings. It makes your diet strategy more sustainable, in short. Remember that it's not just about those first sixteen weeks, but what happens *after*.

For a long-term, sustainable approach, carbs at breakfast, and even throughout the day, just make sense.

The National Weight-Control Registry, which is funded by the National Institute of Health (NIH), is one of the most highly respected studies on long term and sustained weight loss. The registry, established in 1994, has been tracking the eating and diet habits of successful dieters for years. They have tracked thousands and thousands of people confirmed to have lost at least 30 lbs. and kept it off for a year or longer.

One of the most common traits to successful long-term sustainable weight loss that they have observed, according to James Hill, was that, "Almost nobody is on a low-carbohydrate diet." [5]

In fact, these researchers found that the people who were most successful at losing weight and keeping it off were eating high-carbohydrate diets. They usually got about 23% of their calories from fat, which is not too much, but not too little, either.

More broadly, what I'm arguing here is that a successful diet strategy is one of *in*clusion, not *ex*clusion. This means including both starchy carbs like brown rice, potatoes, and oatmeal, and fibrous carbs like bright-coloured vegetables. And sure, a healthy diet strategy will also include fats like whole eggs, healthy oils, natural peanut butter, or raw nuts.

In other words, there are good eating and food strategies to put in place, and there are strategies that are… well, *not* so good to put in place. Unrealistic restrictions (whether they are of total calories, or of a single macronutrient, or they come in the form of a weird cleanse or something) can cause intolerable hunger—the kind of hunger that leads to binging. And, if you last long enough before finally giving in and binging, you can cause metabolic responses that will make things harder down the road.

Instead, as part of your total diet strategy, I recommend eating all three macronutrients. Have a protein at each meal (lean meat, dairy, etc.) and a protein-sparing macronutrient at each meal. This means have either a carb or a fat along with the protein source. However, I recommend that breakfast always use a starchy carb for its protein-sparing macronutrient. Don't worry. In the practical section I'll give you examples of all of this.

I also recommend that you eat healthy whole and unprocessed foods as much as you can, about 90% of the time. This will do wonders for hunger and for getting your satiety feedback systems working as they should so that you can learn to listen to your body and practice real mindful eating. (This is a part of what I mean by integrative fitness and by thinking beyond just "what" you eat.)

Similarly, just as establishing regular meal times is a good diet strategy guideline to follow, establishing regular and consistent sleep and wake times is also a good diet strategy guidelines.

Yes, your sleep absolutely affects your weight and how easy or hard it is to keep weight off. Remember Sylvia from the examples I used at the beginning of this project? She was sleep deprived and didn't establish regular sleep and wake times. She never connected this to her weight issues. By contrast, J.P. works a job that demands irregular sleep. He didn't change his job, but he knew from the get-go that it was a factor, and together we were mindful of it with respect to his hunger, his energy, and his training.

If your answer to this is, "Well, I can't control my sleep times, so I need a diet that takes this into account!" then I'm not explaining myself well.

Let me be more blunt: this or that diet simply *can't* do that, regardless of what it promises.

It just can't.

A real, sustainable diet strategy is one that addresses the whole picture. This doesn't mean you put together a meal plan that somehow can magically overcome the increased hunger that comes with lack of sleep. It means you take into account the hunger that comes with a lack of sleep, and you therefore think about more than just "what" you eat!

Sleep affects hunger, regardless of your diet. It

affects your energy levels, your willpower, and your metabolism. It can be a factor in the release of stress hormones. Can you lose weight while getting poor sleep? Yes, of course that is physiologically possible. But it's harder, and there is no way to get around this. The more one thing like sleep is off, the more you need to have the other things in check (e.g., establishing regular meal times or eating healthy whole foods).

Fad diets don't teach you anything about listening to and connecting with your own body. By following an integrative fitness and diet-strategy approach, by thinking about sleep and recovery, and by not eliminating entire food groups, you will reboot your natural hormones and biochemical processes in a healthy way.

From there you will reestablish what sustainable natural hunger and appetite should feel like. You will start learning from your body.

Your body has wisdom of its own. Hunger, energy, and satiety—these things are your body's way of communicating with you. Don't ignore that wisdom; tap into it!

Diets try to tell you that your body is stupid, and that it's your job as a dieter to just force your body to comply with your restrictions. Wrong. Your body needs to be coaxed, and you need to work with it. If you study high achievers in almost any kind of physical performance, you will see the same pattern over and over again: they trust their body's capabilities and they are able to push themselves because of it. The best athletes know how to listen to their bodies.

Finally, even with all the above said, I want to emphasize that a diet strategy is a mere tool. It's a means of setting things in motion. The magic is not in the diet strategy or the meal plan—not really.

The magic is in *you*. Let me say again: your weight issue is not a diet issue; it is a *you* issue.

Make this about complicated food rules and you will lose. Make it about you, make it about integrative fitness, and make it about emotional self-nurturing and emotional ability, and you will win.

Diet Strategy Tools

I need to comment here about some of the other most common tools used for a healthy diet strategy. Some are useful, some are less useful, and some can be useful or damaging depending on how you use them and think about them.

The Weight Scale

For instance, let's talk about your weight scale. If you can't use a weight scale without attaching *emotional* weight to it, then it serves no purpose for you, at least not for the time being.

A weight scale is a tool, no more and no less. If you can't use it as a simple tool, then don't use it. If you're "afraid" to step on the scale because of what it might show, or if you "dread" the scale, then it just isn't serving you any more.

The weight scale is often a liar, anyway. By contrast, things like how your clothes fit, how you look in your mirror, which belt loop you're using—these things never lie. Remember, we want to get real here. This is not ever going to be about numbers.

Let me put this in perspective: Would you rather a small scale spout a specific arbitrary number, or would you rather fit into those jeans from five or ten years ago? If you just want the number, go buy a scale that shows kilograms instead of pounds. If you want the jeans, follow the approach I'm outlining here.

Numbers can be "indicators," but no more, and even then, that is with the caveat that numbers can lie and not tell you the whole picture.

A scale should never determine your emotional state for the day ahead. It doesn't have that kind of power, except when you *give* it that power.

If you do use a weight scale, it should be used infrequently, not every day or several times per day. If you have a lot of weight to lose, weighing yourself every day only breeds obsession.

My advice is to weigh yourself once per week, on the same day every week, on the same scale every week, and preferably first thing in the morning. Overweight people losing weight can have tremendous water weight fluctuations throughout the day as your body adapts to your diet strategy. Such changes in water weight can be confusing if you are worshipping numbers on the scale. This is why weighing yourself first thing in the morning makes the most sense.

The Food Scale

Now, let's consider food scales, but again, let's consider them as a tool—and no more than that. Food scales come in handy to stay on top of portion sizes. I still use mine and I've been following my diet strategy for decades.

Some food items are hard to "eyeball" in terms of portion sizes, so they are worth measuring out. Usually this means protein sources like meats and fish, and starch sources like oatmeal or potatoes.

At the same time, there are some whole food sources you shouldn't have to measure out. Fresh fruits basically already come in preportioned sizes, and even when they don't, they're not high enough in calories to really warrant the use of a scale. This is even truer for fibrous veggies. The difference between 100 grams and 200 grams of broccoli is nothing, and not worth worrying about. (Hint: As you'll see, your meal plan or strategy should reflect this by not specifying a specific amount for things like fibrous veggies.)

Tolerable Hunger

What I call "tolerable hunger" is an internal tool, if you will. You have to make friends with it. Tolerable hunger gives you important indicators to pay attention to. Tolerable hunger tells you about meal times, and it informs you about your physiological state.

In short: tolerable hunger tells you that you are in a fat-burning mode. This is a good thing! Tolerable hunger means weight loss, and being full or "stuffed" basically stops that weight loss and takes you out of fat-burning mode.

Tolerable hunger should always be just as its name describes: *tolerable*. It should also always come with good physical and mental energy. Indeed, for various physiological reasons, you should actually have better mental energy while you're experiencing tolerable hunger than when you're full.

You don't want to go beyond tolerable hunger into *in*tolerable hunger. Going beyond tolerable hunger to intolerable hunger will likely trigger overeating in the short term and a metabolic down-regulation (slowing of metabolism) in the long term if it goes on for too long before the binge.

You should just "own" living in a state of tolerable hunger. Own the fact that it feels good and it feels better to be neither starved nor stuffed. To be able to live more or less in a state of tolerable hunger means food no longer controls you in any way. It means you control it. You no longer equate being stuffed with being satisfied. You no longer equate tolerable hunger with some kind of deprivation. You simply get real that this level of hunger is sustainable and serves you, mentally, physically, and emotionally.

Accept that of course individual cravings may come and go. But the more you give into them on impulse, the bigger and stronger the craving monster becomes. With tolerable hunger you can tolerate cravings. Just remind yourself, "This too shall pass."

I remember in the early days of my post-professional-bodybuilding years, there were many times when I had to remind myself that my cravings would pass. At first I had to remind myself consistently *not* to feed them or give in to them. This created a physiological habit where the "volume button" for food cravings in my own head just got turned down to practically "mute." My body just learned that I would not feed cravings, so the messages stopped being broadcast. I didn't feed them, which is the number one thing that'll make them grow and intensify.

The one thing you don't want to do is feed your cravings. Make it a habit *not* to feed them. If you give cravings no voice inside your own head, then (surprise!) cravings will no longer have a voice inside your own head.

* * *

This chapter has hopefully given you a better approach or mindset towards a diet strategy.

You'll notice, of course, that there are no specific rules or meal plans here. Don't worry, I *have* included them in the practical section later on in this book where I provide you with a way to construct your own personalized meal plan, and I provide examples of meal plans used by actual clients.

However, I want to stress that it's not about the specific meal plans, except insofar as those plans support everything else. The meal plans should really only reflect how you think about food and weight. They aren't the magic secret. How you use them—that's the secret sauce here.

Chapter References

[4] Jakubowicz, Daniela et al. "Meal Timing and Composition Influence Ghrelin Levels, Appetite Scores and Weight Loss Maintenance in Overweight and Obese Adults." *Steroids* 77.4 (2012): 323–331. Web.

[5] qtd. in Fumento, Michael. "Big Fat Fake: the Atkins Diet Controversy and the Sorry State of Science Journalism." Reason (2003): 1–13. Web.
<http://reason.com/archives/2003/03/01/big-fat-fake/print>

Practical Section

Getting Started

I want to emphasize that embracing integrative fitness and the self-nurturing mindset must come first, before you really dig into any Okay, so you're excited and ready to get started. Good. This section will tell you exactly what to do.

Starting a new diet can be overwhelming. You might also be starting a new exercise program or even starting to exercise for the first time in months or years. On top of that, I've included a number of self-investigation questions.

So, where do you start?

The actions steps in this section are an outline of what you should do in the next few days and over the first week or so.

Most people are excited to get started. Of course, you *should* be excited. But you also don't want to try to do everything at once, burn out, and quit before ever really starting.

There are specific steps I want you to do right away and certain things that can wait. For instance, there are a few steps I want you to take to get your mind right for the journey ahead. Most people jump into the diet and exercise because it feels good to accomplish something, but they neglect really getting their minds right before proceeding.

So, let's set up a working strategy for moving forward—what to do right now and in the week ahead.

The First Day or Two:

- To set your mind right, go to the questionnaire and self-investigation section and do the first few "Getting Started" questions. There are a lot of questions, so you don't have to do all of them at once, but do the first three in that Getting Started section. (Get a pen and paper and write them out. Later, perhaps when you go grocery shopping, you might consider picking up a cheap notebook for some of the other ones.)

- Take a look at the meal plan examples. Familiarize yourself with them. Pick one to use as a starting point and just get started. Follow the guidelines for any of them, and you really can't go wrong. Remind yourself to stick to healthy whole foods and use these diets as "examples" that you can personalize from there.

- Take a look at the exercise section below and the programs provided and maybe decide which program is for you based on the overview at the beginning of that section. **You don't have to start exercising today or tomorrow.** I want you to just look at the program and familiarize yourself with whichever one you choose. Maybe use Google to search for exercises you don't know, or look for them in my exercise library at scottabelfitness.com/library. (I've tried to be exhaustive, but if there are some you don't know and they don't show up in the first few results in Google, email me.)

- Take a few days to a week to continue to look these things over, rather than feel a need to jump in and get started "right now." My point is simply to *slow down*. Familiarize yourself with these things. Take the attitude of "no pressure." The trick is to ease into the process, and become comfortable *with* that process.

From there, everything else will fall into place.

The First Week:

- Make an attempt to cook some meals and start to think about logistics. You don't have to be perfect at first. You'll learn what works as you go, but preparing at least some meals in advance for the week ahead is something every single fit and healthy person I know does on a regular basis. At the same time, everyone is different when it comes to individual logistics; there's nothing to do except feel it out and find out what works for your schedule.

- When you've selected your meal plan, go grocery shopping for what you need. Get in the habit of doing it and enjoying it. Don't leave it to someone else. Get in the habit of doing it *before* you've run out of something. (Again, you might not be perfect with this at first. That's fine. You'll work things out as you go.) Shop ahead, prepare ahead. This is something you can also start this week.

- Maybe try to start the exercise plan, even if

it is just the first workout. Feel it out and have fun with it. Or if your plan involves just walking, plan out a route in Google Maps or something. (Or, alternatively, enjoy exploring, with no plan at all.) For now, it doesn't matter how long you go. Just put yourself out there and try it.

- Start going over some of the *other* self-investigation questions if you have time. Try to make it a habit to do a few every few days, and maybe start journaling. That's up to you, as everyone is different.

What to Expect After Your First Week

Are you ready for this?

Expect NOTHING.

The best way to truly immerse yourself in the process is to stop with all the false expectations. Remember, do *not* make this about super fast, "want-it-now" weight loss. You have to make it about lifestyle and the process.

You don't sit around with expectations after showering in the morning or taking your garbage out. This is all about creating a lifestyle and a set of habits that serve you.

For the first week, the action steps above are

enough. **Don't expect any weight loss at all. It will come, I promise. (I've been at this a long, long time.) But for now, the process is what matters.**

If you don't hit all your meals at first, that's fine. If you go grocery shopping but forget something, and you can't make all your meals, well, *that's fine too!* You'll fix it next time. Focus on the process and the rest will come.

Don't overwhelm yourself. This is no longer about looking for magic in diets or having expectations that create anxiety in you. Just work the program and the program will work. This is all about learning to be patient and investing in the process until it becomes a lifestyle.

Allow the plan do its work. Don't try to fix things and change things right from the beginning. Start looking for insights (how you feel emotionally, how tolerable hunger feels, how your energy is doing) rather than looking for "out-sights" (like how many calories you burned or how much weight you lost). This first week is all about "getting acquainted."

Let that be your only expectation.

Your Diet Strategy and Meal Plan

Many people confuse letting go of the North American diet mentality with having no diet strategy at all and eating according to whim and instinct. That is not necessarily the point. Having some structure and regimentation here can be helpful, without it being a prison.

Remember the old Buddhist expression from the introduction:

"Before enlightenment, I chopped wood and carried water; after enlightenment, I chopped wood and carried water."

Letting go of the diet mentality doesn't mean you can't have any planned or scheduled meals anymore. That has never been the argument.

You just don't make it about doing "this diet" or "that diet." You create a plan that works for you. You choose to follow an eating strategy based on self-nurturing, on getting real, and on truly integrative fitness.

You can and should still follow some kind of regimented eating plan like the ones below. However, the mindset that drives it should be very, very different.

You'll see the examples are from my own clients, though I've included information and strategies to personalize them or create your own. This is all done within the mental framework of choosing healthy whole foods.

Again, don't feel like you have to dive into a diet strategy with the "cold turkey" approach. That may not work for you.

You may at first just want to do one or two of the diet meals per day for a week to a few weeks. (Perhaps try to swap them in for the meals you know are currently serving you "least.")

This will give you time and mental energy to work your way into the whole diet. You start with a couple of the healthy meals listed, but you also keep some of your own meals for a bit. Eventually, you can add in another healthy meal from the diet when you feel ready. My clients often have success with this approach because it makes the mind feel that there is more "choice" involved rather than pressure and deprivation.

A Quick Word about Cheat Meals:

So common are cheat days and refeed days now in the diet world that people ask me about them all the time, partly because I've been using them for 30+ years, and I even have a diet based on cheat days and refeeds called the Cycle Diet. *However,* if we're being real, then know that if you have 20, 30, 40 or more pounds to lose, there is no way you need to be planning "refeeds." If you have a lot of weight to lose, and you're on a reasonable diet (like the ones below), then metabolically there is no reason to have them.

Having said that, I've said several times that you aren't expected to be some kind of diet zombie either. There will be times when getting away from your diet strategy just serves to reboot your commitment to it again. Every so often, in an unscheduled way, have a meal that's not part of your diet strategy. Just don't use this as an excuse to have an off-diet meal every other day or all weekend because it's just too hard without the structure of your workday. These are not get-real mindsets.

Instead, have a meal that is not part of the diet strategy every now and then. Accept it for what it is. It doesn't "make you a failure," but on the other end of the spectrum, that doesn't mean you "deserve" it because it's Friday and you had a hard week. It's *just food*, and you are a human being.

Maybe it's an important occasion. Maybe you've just been craving a certain meal for two weeks and you want to indulge, and you have a mature mindset and you know that it won't throw off your entire diet.

Portion Sizes

Now, portion sizes. There are some things worth measuring in portion sizes, and other things not really worth measuring at all. Instead of giving complicated caloric formulas, it's actually safe to skip all that and just stick to reasonable portion sizes on a per meal basis.

I'll mention normal portion sizes here just to give you an idea.

Women:

- Animal protein sources and meats: 90-120 grams precooked weight.
- Egg whites: 200-250 mls
- Whole eggs: 1-2
- Raw nuts: 20-30 grams
- Healthy fats: 1/2-1 tbsp.
- Starches like rice: 1/4-1/3 cup (cooked weight)
- Oats and related dry cereals: 1/4-1/3 cup dry weight
- Potatoes, sweet potatoes, etc.: 100-120 grams by weight, precooked.
- I don't really see a need to measure whole fruits or fibrous veggies. Use condiments for taste, in moderation.

Men:

- Animal protein sources and meats: 120-150 grams precooked weight
- Egg whites: 250 mls
- Whole eggs: 2-3

- Raw nuts: 40-50 grams
- Healthy fats: 1-2 tbsp.
- Starches like rice: 1/3–1 cup (cooked weight)
- Oats and related dry cereals: 1/2 – 2/3 cups dry weight
- Potatoes, sweet potatoes, etc.: choose small to medium size or 120–180 grams by weight, precooked.
- Again, as with women, I don't really see a need to measure whole fruits or fibrous veggies. Use condiments for taste, in moderation.

This is just a very general way to keep portion sizes controlled within metabolically supportive limits without getting all caught up again in calorie-counting madness.

How Do I Know the "Right" Portion Size to Pick If There is Such a Variance in Choice?

There is no "right" choice! When you use portion sizes without any calorie-counting nonsense, you become more in touch with your own internal mechanisms for hunger and satiety.

Remember "tolerable hunger" is the goal and the sweet spot where you want to stay 90% of the time. By eliminating calorie counting, you get back to using your own subjective assessment of "tolerable hunger," based on the portion sizes you choose.

Now, I have had clients have major success by taking two initial starting strategies.

Many clients who have lost a lot of weight only to gain it all back "fear" being too hungry following any given diet strategy. For such clients, I always suggest they start with the maximum portion sizes listed. Most of them initially find this to be too much food, so they don't experience "tolerable hunger" at first, but it does help them get over the fear of being too hungry. From there, they just gradually cut portions bit by bit, coaxing their bodies towards a tolerable, reasonable, and maintainable amount of hunger (with good energy). If they find their sweet spot for tolerable hunger somewhere between the maximum allowable portions and the minimum, then they have found their way to a sustainable diet-strategy lifestyle that is still individualized.

I've had other clients achieve equal success by taking the exact opposite approach—they just opt for the lower portions! They're not too afraid of being hungry. By starting from the lower end, they know that they can eat more if needed, and if hunger edges towards being *in*tolerable, they know they definitely do "need" to increase their portion sizes. At this point, it's no longer about eating more just because they want to, but because they're finally listening to their bodies. Many of them also find that this approach allows them to eat more as they lose weight and they are able to walk further, walk faster, work out harder, and so on. Then they can gradually work towards eating the maximum portion sizes listed—*if they need to*! If they don't need to eat the larger portions based on assessing their tolerable hunger, they stay where they are.

Simply using portion sizes is better than the endless number crunching of counting each calorie. Counting calories always misleads you; it provides the illusion of control, not *actual* control. Metabolism is about much more than energy in, energy out. By using portion sizes in relation to assessing your own tolerable hunger, you are working "with" your body and "with" your metabolism in a more integrated kind of way.

Example Male Diet
JP

This is the diet that my client JP used for his remarkable transformation you saw in the introduction.

Meal 1

- 8 egg whites (250 mls) or 2–3 whole eggs (egg whites preferred).
- 2/3 cup dry weight (about 55-60g) of cream of wheat, oatmeal, or oat bran, or other hot cereal. Can also sub 3 large shredded wheat biscuits.

Meal 2

- 40–50 grams raw nuts (either almonds, walnuts, peanuts or pecans).
- 2/3 cup cooked quinoa or buckwheat groats, or 2/3 cup brown rice mixed with 1 cup or so fibrous veggies, and 6–8 oz. tomato juice or one large pickle optional if you don't have veggies in the rice.

Meal 3

- 40–50 grams raw nuts as above, or 1 1/2 cups 1% cottage cheese.

- 3 pieces or equivalent of fresh fruit. (e.g., One piece would be 1 large banana, 1 large apple, 1 large orange, or 2 cups mixed berries. No need to measure.)

Meal 4

- 120-150g chicken breast or 1 can tuna, or 8 egg whites, or 120g red meat.

- 1/2–2/3 cup cooked rice with 1–2 cups vegetables, like green beans or yellow beans etc., anything except peas or corn.

Meal 5

- 120–150g chicken or turkey breast, or 1 can tuna packed in water.

- Medium to large salad, vinegar, 1–2 tbsp. extra virgin olive oil (all salad ingredients allowed), small to medium size potato or yam.

General Guidelines

- Meal 5 can sub 1 cup cooked peas instead of salad, and 2/3 cup cooked rice instead of yam/potato.

- The word "or" at any of the above meals means choose one of the options given (for protein or carbs etc.) and only one.

- All weights precooked weight unless otherwise stated. But feel free to switch the order of the meals around; they do not have to be consumed in this exact order

- Once per day, 2–3 cups mixed veggies, frozen or fresh, can be subbed for carbs at any meal. If you do this, add 1–2 tbps. extra virgin olive oil or any healthy oil to the salad (canola, coconut, macadamia, flax).

- Condiments are fine, in moderation. Stick mainly to mustard, ketchup, relish, salsa, hot sauce, non-fat mayo, or any of the low-calorie dressings for your salad, artificial sweetener. The key is "in moderation." And if you're not sure of a condiment, don't use it.

- Once or twice per week a good meal option is a large salad composed of baby spinach, as much as you want, kale, cucumber, peppers, other salad ingredients, add in 1 tbsp. dried cranberry, 1 tbsp. pumpkin or flax seeds, 2/3 cups chickpeas, with extra virgin olive oil and balsamic vinegar (not store bought "vinaigrette").

- It's okay to cook things like buckwheat groats or quinoa in a small amount of vegetable broth (not oil) with the water (as part of the liquid measurement).

- Any whitefish or even salmon steak can be subbed for protein source at meal 4 or meal 5.

- If you do not care for fish, then instead of tuna you can sub in 120 grams of flank steak, inside round steak, or pork tenderloin, but only once per week.

- Meals should always be kept 3–4 hours apart.

- Never combine meals, and all meal are interchangeable in terms of order.

- Coffee and tea are fine, as is diet soda, but keep that to a minimum. Aim for as much water as you can drink for the majority of your fluid needs.

Example Female Diet Alba

This is the exact diet that my client Alba used for her transformation.

Meal 1

- 4–8 egg whites (125-250 mls)
- 60g dry weight of oatmeal, cream of wheat, oat bran or other dry cereal. Add 1tbsp. flaxseed.

OR

- 1 cup plain non-fat Greek yogurt with fresh fruit that YOU add (i.e., don't get the stuff where it's already mixed in, because they add other things). No need to measure. Can also add 1 tbsp. Macadamia nut oil or flax seeds.

OR

- 1 or 2 whole eggs, cooked any style you prefer.
- 1–2 slices of Ezekiel bread and 1 tbsp. natural peanut butter or almond butter.

Meal 2

- 90–100g cooked whitefish, OR 100g of chicken breast or turkey breast, OR 8 egg whites.
- 1 small to medium potato or yam, plus 1–2 cups of cooked veggies with 1–2 tbsp. extra virgin olive oil.

Meal 3

- 100g chicken or turkey breast, OR 30g raw nuts.
- 3 large rice cakes (any flavour except sweet ones like "caramel"), OR 1 small to medium potato or yam, OR 1/4–1/2 cups of cooked brown rice, plus any fibrous veggies you'd prefer, cooked with 1 tbsp. extra virgin olive oil.

Meal 4

- 90–120 grams any whitefish OR 90–100 grams chicken or turkey breast.
- 1 small to medium potato or yam, OR 2/3 cup cooked rice, any kind, with small salad with low-calorie dressing for taste.

OR

- 30–40 grams any unsalted raw nuts, OR 2/3 cup 1% cottage cheese.
- 2–3 pieces of any fresh fruit you'd like, no need to measure.

Meal 5

- 100–120g fish or 8 egg whites (250 mls).
- 1/4–1/2 cooked brown or basmati or jasmine rice with either some fibrous veggies or a small salad with 1 tbsp. olive oil.

General Guidelines

- All weights are precooked unless otherwise indicated.
- The word "or" at any of the above meals, means choose one of the options given (for protein, or carbs etc.) and only one.
- Once or twice per week, red meat, in the form of flank steak, inside round steak, extra lean ground beef, or pork tenderloin can be had in place of any protein source above. Aim for about 120 grams

precooked weight.

- An optional meal to sub for any of the above would be regular salad ingredients with about 1/3 cup chickpeas or edamame for protein. Add some pumpkin seeds or sunflower seeds (or hemp seeds, flax seeds), and maybe a bit of feta cheese and some dried cranberries. Add balsamic vinegar or low-calorie dressing.

- Quinoa can be subbed in place of rice or oats at any time. Aim for about 60 grams dry weight of quinoa.

- Where I indicate "fibrous veggies," that just means green or yellow beans, squash, peppers (green, red, yellow), mushrooms, radish, asparagus, broccoli, cauliflower—any of them, really. Some find that mixing a lot of fibrous veggies gives them a bit of gas. If that's the case, choose just one of your choice, or use one of the other options (usually a small salad).

- For condiments, you can use ketchup, mustard, chili ketchup, salsa, hot sauces, any artificial sweeteners, spices, non-fat mayo, low-calorie salad dressings, and so on.

- Meals should always be kept 3–4 hours

apart.

- Never combine meals, and all meal are interchangeable in terms of order.
- Coffee and tea are fine, as is diet soda, but keep that to a minimum. Aim for as much water as you can drink for the majority of your fluid needs.

The Best Whole Food Sources

Below is a quick reference for healthy whole food sources.

If something is not on this list below, then it is not likely a healthy whole food choice. So let's focus on what is good and helpful and will provide satiety, energy, and a variety of tastes and textures.

Healthy Animal Flesh Protein Sources

- Boneless skinless chicken breast, boneless skinless turkey breast, extra lean ground beef, extra lean ground chicken or turkey.

- Fish, such as tuna packed in water (albacore is the best), plus any variations of whitefish including orange roughy,

halibut, haddock, cod, sole, flounder, whitefish, salmon, trout, sea bass, pickerel.
- Shellfish choices like shrimp and scallops.
- Red meats like flank steak, inside round, buffalo or bison, pork tenderloin, any wild game meats.
- Generally, red meat and shellfish choices should be limited to once or twice per week.

Other Healthy Protein Sources

- Low-fat or non-fat cottage cheese, low-fat or non-fat plain yogurt.
- Raw unsalted nuts, natural nut butters, raw unsalted seeds.
- Whey protein should be used in moderation. It is still generally considered "a processed food," but of course it is convenient sometimes. Real whole foods from real sources are always the better choice.

Healthy Starchy Carb Sources

- Oatmeal, oat bran, shredded wheat

biscuits (the kind without frosting!), grits, cream of rice cereal, cream of wheat cereal.

- Brown rice, jasmine rice, basmati rice, wild rice. The longer rice takes to cook, the better.

- Yams, potatoes (any kind), sweet potatoes, peas.

- Rice cakes, rice chips, or "minis"—large and small. Any flavour except the sweet ones are okay, but no more than once per day, mostly for convenience.

Fibrous Veggies

- Carrots, spinach, mushrooms, kale, spinach, asparagus, squash, peppers (red, yellow or green), green or yellow string beans, snap peas, cabbage, broccoli, cauliflower, eggplant, zucchini, beets, Brussels sprouts, turnip, pumpkin, lettuce. Pretty much all fibrous veggies are allowed and encouraged.

- Frozen veggies mixes are also allowed and encouraged.

Fruits

- Apples, oranges, pears, grapefruit, strawberries, blueberries, pineapples, cherries, raspberries, cantaloupe, grapes, mangoes, bananas, peaches.

- All raw natural fruits are allowed and encouraged.

Healthy Fats

- Extra virgin olive oil (sometimes abbreviated EVOO), extra virgin coconut oil, flax oil, macadamia nut oil, canola oil.

- Raw nuts, nut butters, and so on, are also good, and will also contain a bit of protein.

General Condiments

(To use in moderation for taste or for cooking.)

- Cooking spray
- Herbs and spices (preferably not the salt forms)
- Mustard
- Ketchup
- Red hot sauce, any hot sauce

- Salsa
- Any artificial sweetener
- Lite, low-sodium soy sauce
- Fat-free or calorie-wise or light salad dressings
- Low-fat or non-fat mayo
- Generally, most condiments that are low in calorie and don't contain and lot of sugar are okay *in moderation*. With my coaching clients, I usually have them ask me, but mostly the answer is "yes, in moderation."

Fluids

- Of course, water is always the best fluid choice! (Drinking calories isn't optimal for things like satiety.)
- Almost all diet drinks are fine in moderation. In general do not "drink" your calories; therefore calorie-free diet drinks are recommended
- Tea and coffee are just fine. Use artificial sweetener for them, and a little dash or milk or cream is okay too. (Again, in moderation.)

Your Exercise Plan

Keep this in mind regarding getting real with your desire to lose substantial weight and keep it off. You are not going to do this through diet *alone*. Not long term, at least.

The benefits of exercise for your body's overall health—and for your soul and self-connection—extend far beyond "burning calories." This is especially true as you get older.

At the highest levels, exercise becomes something greater than itself. You lose yourself and find yourself at the same time. Instead of a source of energy drain and exhaustion, it becomes a source of energy renewal, invigoration, and inspiration.

The old adage I like to use here is, "Real winners forget they are even in a race; real winners just love to run."

Walking

If you're very overweight, or if it's been years since you stepped inside a gym, then my absolute number one preferred exercise strategy for you is simply to get walking. Aside from its other benefits, walking is a wonderful way to develop mindfulness. It has wonderful cognitive and emotional benefits that can help you straighten out your thoughts, especially if you sometimes feel overwhelmed or overloaded.

Walking is also easy to do. All it takes is a comfortable pair of shoes. You can walk wherever you feel most comfortable. It's not something you need to "learn" or spend money investing in before you can get started. If you're travelling, you don't need to find a gym. You can do it in the morning, at lunch, or whenever feels best for you.

On the physical fitness and metabolism side of the exercise equation I prefer walking for several reasons. The first is that it is just so natural for all of us. Next, it gets you standing as you move your body—you're not sitting down or strapped into a machine.

Also, let's not forget, if you are carrying around a substantial amount of excess weight, then this extra weight you carry is systemically a metabolic stimulus when you're walking and carrying it around. Walking with a lot of excess weight is a lot like wearing a weighted vest for everything you do. The "resistance" is already there, "on" your body.

Walking is less likely to lead to injuries or to wear and tear on hips, knees, and lower back. When you are overweight, it is very easy to strain these areas if you try things like running.

I have written a lot in the past about "the aerobic myth" for fat loss and leaning out, but most of it does not apply if you have substantial weight to lose. The benefits of it are increased, and the drawbacks are negligible. You are carrying around enough added resistance in the form of extra weight that walking can serve you well.

You don't need to make a walking protocol complicated. You don't need to worry about "intervals" or "HIIT." You don't need to measure your speed. If you only have ten minutes, then walk for ten minutes. I will suggest more below when it comes to a full exercise program, but the mindset of doing it when you can, and doing it to feel better, is just as important. Keep it simple… and walk! If it's nasty outside then walk on a treadmill. Just walk.

That old phrase, *The longest journey begins with a single step,* can be really embraced here, both literally and metaphorically.

Adding in a Resistance Program

At some point, you will want to incorporate resistance training. You don't have to do it right when you get started, but almost assuredly, at some point it will be a huge step forward for you, if you're not doing any resistance training at all right now. Resistance training has tremendous carryover in terms of positive metabolic effects as you move forward and drop weight.

Now, many of you may be at different levels of fitness. You may have physical limitations because of your weight. You may have medical issues because of your weight that cause physical limitations with exercise as well. (Note that as you lose weight, you tend to need less and less medication—at least the kinds of medications that are the direct result of your weight.)

Therefore, other than the above prescription for walking, I am leery of assigning a "one-size-fits-all" program. However, with that said, I have used the two programs below for decades to help clients who've had substantial weight to lose.

These programs, combined with cardiovascular work as simple as walking, are all you really need to get you started. Could you start a new program a few months down the line? Sure. If you lose a lot of weight, it is likely you'll want to. But programs like that are easy enough to find. For now, get started with a program like the two you see here.

These two programs below are "whole body programs," and they are meant to be done by beginners, two or three times per week. If you're just getting started, start with twice per week; if you are not a beginner, then three times per week is optimal.

These workouts are meant to be done on *nonconsecutive* days. So don't work out Monday, Tuesday, Wednesday and then take the rest of the week off. Always have a day of rest in between each workout. If that means one week you only work out twice instead of three times, that's okay.

This means if you do Workout 1 on a Monday, you are not going to do Workout 2 until at *least* Wednesday.

Of course, you can walk as much as you want, for as long as you want, on any day of the week, whether you work out on that day or not. Walking will not tap into your recovery; if anything, it might help, and it will definitely enhance your overall fitness moving forward. If you want, you can also add some walking to the end of each of these workouts if you have the time. Anywhere from 10 to 30 minutes of walking or cardio can be done immediately after finishing these workouts.

On in-between days from weight training, I suggest walking or mixing up nonballistic cardio exercise (e.g., going for a bike ride) for anywhere from 35 to 60 minutes. If you have the time and the desire, a leisurely walk for up to two hours would be fine as well. Don't make it about intensity and exhaustion; leave that nonsense to Hollywood and reality TV. Make it about consistency and something you can and want to do regularly.

The Programs

(The application instructions here are for both Program A and Program B)

These programs are considered "start" programs. Many of you who are overweight but exercise regularly may be just fine doing your own current workout programs if you enjoy them.

But these programs below are for those of you starting an exercise regimen or getting back to one after a long layoff because of your weight.

If you were incorporating some walking and

maybe a few other nonballistic forms of cardio when you had the chance, then a typical week may look something like this:

- **Monday: <u>Workout #1</u>**
- **Tuesday:** A walk outside during lunch.
- **Wednesday:** Walk on treadmill for a while, then ride stationary bike for a bit of time.
- **Thursday: <u>Workout #2</u>**, followed by ten minutes on the treadmill.
- **Friday:** A walk outside after work.
- **Saturday:** Walk on treadmill for a while, then ride stationary bike for a bit of time.
- **Sunday:** Off.

The above is *not* a strict prescription. It's just an example from one of my previous clients with a busy schedule, and how he fit in his workouts and his walking and cardio sessions. Later on, he might have tried to fit in three resistance-training workouts per week and removed one of his walking sessions.

It's nothing complicated and he made use of the time and energy he had. So again, just keep it simple and keep it doable. Don't overreach. Overreaching has never likely worked for you before.

Program Guidelines

- Try to choose a weight where you are challenged for the reps indicated. (Except the first set, which serves as a warm up). But do *not* train to the point where you can't finish the last rep. This is called "training to failure."

- Move at your own pace from set to set, and from exercise to exercise.

- Rest long enough between sets that you can subjectively determine that you can perform the next set with equal intensity. Do *not* rush. You should never be panting when you start the next set. Eventually your pace will get faster on its own as you condition into the program. This happens with every program.

- This slash symbol "/" between two exercises means superset the two exercises as one. So I might write, "Tubing or cable pulldowns / SB Hip Bridges." That means you do them back to back without rest for the reps indicated, and then you will take normal post-set rest after completion of the second exercise. On the next set (or superset), you do both of them again.

- Workouts should be completed within 45-60 minutes or so.

- Train two or three days per week, on nonconsecutive days.

- Go completely through the full set of workouts for the program, then just start from the beginning. It might take you a week and a half to go through them for Program A, or it might take two weeks and a bit for Program B. The workouts are not linked to specific days of the week. Once you reach the end, you just go back to the beginning for your next workout.

- Program should be done in straight sets with adequate recovery between sets and no sets performed to failure.

- Hammer grip just means arms at your sides to begin and finish, so palms face the side of each leg.

- Follow the workouts in order and then repeat from the beginning. Continue to repeat this cycle for at least three months.

Key

Alt. = Alternate
BB = Barbell
DB = Dumbbell
SB = Stability Ball
MB = Medicine Ball
BW = Bodyweight
M = Max
EL = Each Leg
EA = Each Arm
ES = Each Side
EW = Each Way

Workout Program A

All exercises are listed in the format:

	Sets	Reps
Exercise Name	2	15-20

Sometimes you will see something like:

	Sets	Reps
Exercise Name	3	10, 12, 12-15

In this example, that just means for the first set do 10 reps, for the second set do 12 reps, and for the third set do between 12 and 15 reps.

These are not circuit workouts. That means you do each exercise one at a time. So, for example, in Workout 1, you will start by doing three sets of Leg Press before moving on to the Lying Leg Curls.

WORKOUT 1

	Sets	Reps
Leg Press	3	15-20
Lying Leg Curls	3	20, 15, 20
Hack Squats or DB Squats	1	20
Seated Rows	2	15, 12
Bentover Rows	1	12-15
Machine Shoulder Press	3	15, 12, 10
DB or BB Upright Rows	2	15, 10-12
Machine Chest Press	3	8-10
Flat DB Flyes	2	15, 10-12
DB Concentration Curls	1	15-20
Standing Barbell Curls	1	10-12
Triceps Pushdowns	2	10-12
1-Arm DB Extension	1	10-12

WORKOUT 2

	Sets	Reps
BW or DB squats	3	25, 20, 15
Leg Extensions	2	15-20
1-Arm DB Rows	3	8-10
Lat Pulldowns	2	12-15
Incline DB Press	2	15, 12
"Pec dec" or Chest Fly Machine	1	15-20
Seated Side Laterals	3	15, 12, 10
Alternate DB Press (shoulder)	1	12-15
Overhead Rope Extensions	1	12-15
One-Arm Preacher Curls	1	8-10
Sit-ups of any kind	1	12-15

WORKOUT 3

	Sets	Reps
Leg Press or Hack Squats	3	20, 15, 10-12
Alternating Lunges	2	10-12 EL
DB Stiff-Legged Deadlift	1	12-15
Flat DB Bench Press	3	8-12
Incline Press Machine or DB press	1	12-15
Seated Cable Rows	3	15, 12, 10
Reverse Grip Pulldowns*	1	10-12
Bent DB Lateral Raises	2	12-15
Front DB Alternate Raises	1	12-15 EA
Lying DB or BB Triceps Extensions	2	12-15
Standing BB or Cable Curls	2	10-15
Triceps Pushdowns	1	10-15
DB Concentration Curls	1	10-12

Reverse Grip means palms facing towards you.

WORKOUT 4

	Sets	Reps
Leg Extensions	3	20, 15, 10
Leg Curls	3	15, 12, 10
1-Legged Press	1	15-20
Incline BB or Incline Machine Press	2	8-12
Seated Machine or Cable Flyes	1	8-10
1-Arm DB Rows	1	8-10
Close Grip Pulldowns	2	10-12
Machine Shoulder Press	3	15, 12, 10
Bent DB Laterals	1	15-20
1-Arm DB Extensions	1	10-15
Incline Alternate DB Curls	1	8-10
Standing BB Curls	1	10-12
1-Arm Pushdowns	1	12-15

Workout Program B

As with Workout Program A, all exercises are listed in the format:

	Sets	Reps
Exercise Name	4	15-20

Sometimes you will see something like this:

	Sets	Reps
Exercise / Another Exercise	2	15-20 / 8-10

This just means a super set. You do the first exercise for 15-20 reps, then immediately do the second one for 8-10 reps. You rest, as you normally do between sets then do the second set of each.

Program B is a *slightly* more advanced program than Program A. Just make sure to ease into it, follow the application instructions, and you'll be fine.

WORKOUT 1

	Sets	Reps
DB Squats or hack squats	4	15-20
DB or BW Military Burpees (with or without jump)	3	10-12
DB or MB Vertical Choppers	2	12-15
Recline Pull-Ups, any kind	2	12-15
Seated DB Shoulder Press	2	12-15
DB or BB Bent Rows	2	10-12
Reverse Grip Pulldowns	2	10-12
MB or DB Alt Lateral Reach Lunge and Push	2	10-15 ES
Lying Triceps Extension, DB or BB	2	2 X 12-15
Cable or Tubing Concentration Curls	2	2 X 12-15
Overhead DB Lockout Holds	2	slow 30 count

WORKOUT 2

	Sets	Reps
Leg Press / Leg Curls (any kind)*	4	15-20 / 10-12
Bulgarian Split Squats, DB or BB	3	10-12 EL
Single Leg Step Ups into Reverse Lunge	2	8-12 EL
Incline Barbell or Incline DB Press	2	10-12
Bent DB Laterals	2	12-15
Tubing or Cable Pulldowns / SB Hip Bridges*	2	12-15 / 12-15
SB Straight leg Lateral Raises	2	12-15 ES
Alt. DB Side Laterals, with a contralateral front step**	2	12-15 ES
DB Squat / Hammer Curl and Press	2	15-20
Overhead Tubing or Overhead Rope Triceps Extension	2	12-15
Standing Barbell Curls	2	10-12

This slash symbol / means superset the two listed exercises and do them together back to back without rest, then take a normal rest after completion of the second exercise.

** Contralateral means "opposite side of." So if you raise the dumbbell with your left hand, you step with your right foot.

WORKOUT 3

	Sets	Reps
DB Curl and Press	4	15-20
Leg Press	3	20-25
Machine or Tubing Chest Press (any kind)	2	10-12
DB Upright Rows	2	15-20
Seated Cable Rows	2	12-15
Tubing or Cable Squat with Row	2	12-15
Standing 2-Arm DB Shoulder Press (split stance)	2	12-15
Seated Triceps 1-Arm DB Extension	2	12-15
Alternate Hammer Curls	2	12-15
Low to High Choppers with Tubing or Cables	2	12-15 ES
SB Alternating Step Offs	2	12-15 EL

WORKOUT 4

	Sets	Reps
Barbell or DB Deadlifts*	4	8-10
DB or BW Lunges (alternating legs)	3	12-15 EL
Diamond Push-Ups on Floor or MB (short ROM is fine)	2	8-15
Flat DB Flyes	2	12-15
Alternating Overhead DB Press, seated	2	12-15 ES
1-Arm DB Rows	2	12-15
Seated Cable Rows	2	10-12
DB Alternate Hammer** Curl and Press	2	10-12 EA
DB Side Lateral Throws	2	12-15 EA
Front Alternate DB Raises	2	10-15
Alt. DB Curls or Alt. Hammer Curls	2	10-12 EA

* *Never go even <u>close</u> to failure on deadlifts*

** *"Hammer" just means palms facing inwards (hold the dumbbell as you would if it were a hammer).*

WORKOUT 5

	Sets	Reps
Hack Squats or Any Squat Machine	4	15-20
BW Single Leg Burpees	3	5-8 EL
MB or DB Alt Front Reach Lunge with Overhead Press	2	12-15 ES
Any Seated Chest Press Variation	2	12-15
Reverse Grip Pulldown / Seated Alternate DB Curls *	2	15-20 / 10-12
Standing 1-Arm Tubing or Cable Rows	2	10-12
One-Arm DB Snatch from Hang	2	6-8 EA
One-Arm DB Swings to Front, heavy	2	10-12 EA
Machine or Tubing Preacher Curls	2	10-12
2-Arm Triceps Pushdown	2	12-15
BW One-Legged Glutes Bridges from Floor	2	15-25 EL

This slash symbol / means superset the two listed exercises and do them together back to back without rest, then take a normal rest after completion of the second exercise.

WORKOUT 6

	Sets	Reps
Leg Press or DB Squats	4	15-20
DB or BW Burpee (with or without a jump)	3	8-10
DB Posterior Reaching Lunge with Upright Row*	2	10-12 ES
Incline DB Press / Leg Extensions*	2	10-12 / 12-15
Any Push-ups Variation	2	10-12
DB Upright Rows	2	10-12
Shoulder Press, any kind	2	12-15
Machine Chest Flyes or Cable Crossovers	2	12-15
High to Low Tubing or Cable Chopper	2	12-15
Lying Triceps Extension / SB Hyperextensions	2	12-15 / 12-15
SB Skiers or Side Plank Holds	2	15-20 ES or slow 30 count

* *Use relatively light dumbbells.*

** *This slash symbol / means superset the two listed exercises and do them together back to back without rest, then take a normal rest after completion of the second exercise.*

Self-Investigation Section

This questionnaire and self-investigation section is meant to help you piece together where and how you may be stuck with respect to your weight issue. This whole project takes a mindfulness and a self-awareness approach to weight loss. These exercises lead you in the direction of positive, permanent change. You will find answers to these questions to be very self-revealing.

The questionnaires and exercises below are easy to do and fairly quick to get through. Do them at your own pace. You will see they line up fairly well with the various sections in this book.

(I'll also note that you'll find that very "simple" answers can be lead-ins for you to expand on in your own journaling, something which I highly recommend.)

Keep in mind that the actual content of each answer is less important than the fact that simply asking yourself these questions and then addressing them directly brings all sorts of things up into your conscious awareness. Focus on the questions that resonate with you most—not necessarily in a good or a bad way, but in a "holy crap" way.

Some of the questions below are modified from exercises in Geneen Roth's *Why Weight? A Guide to End Compulsive Eating* (1989) and Tracy Gaudet's *Consciously Female: How to Listen to Your Body and Soul for a Lifetime of Healthy Living* (2004). I recommend both these books heartily.

Getting Started Questions

These questions should be done in the first few days, before you really dig down and get started with a diet strategy or exercise program.

Exercise 1.

This first one is based very directly on a question from Geneen Roth's book (page 44 of my edition). To begin, make a list of all the diets you've ever been on. Try to name them. Go through everything you've tried in the past. Start with the most recent and just work backwards from there. If you have trouble remembering, or they they don't all come to mind in order, don't worry, just do what you can. (Also, if you've done so many that you can't remember them all, that should tell you something!)

Once you've got a list, go through and make some notes on the following:

1. What did you eat and *not* eat on those diets? What were the "food rules?"
2. Did you lose weight?
3. How long did you keep it off before weight started creeping back on?
4. How long did you sustain the diet as a lifestyle?
5. How much weight did you gain when you went off the diet?
6. Did your appetite and hunger change as a result of this diet? If so, how?
7. What does answering these questions tell you about this specific diet?

As you go, you might also add in your own comments, journaling style. Were you frustrated on the diet, or did you enjoy the diet at first? What happened? What didn't work? Why couldn't you sustain it? How do you feel about the diet now?

Once you're done, look at this whole list and ask yourself, "If diets really worked for me in taking weight off and keeping it off, then why do

I end up going on so many of them?" Try to write as long and as detailed a response as you can to this.

Remember, a diet that works for you is a diet strategy that you can sustain forever *without* putting the weight back on. If it can't sustain it, or if the weight comes back, then by definition, that diet *did not work*.

Exercise 2.

What do you judge negatively about yourself, especially with respect to your own weight?

Make a full list of all the kinds of things you say to yourself regarding your weight, your attempts at dieting, and anything else related to these things.

Once that's done, ask yourself, what does this tell you about your mindset? Then, take a look at what you've written and consider how you can frame things more positively. Take a glance at the "Semantic Sanity" section in the chapter on Karl Albrecht's Four Mental Habits to Increase Mental Productivity for examples of reframing your self-talk. How can you make these statements more empowering and useful to you? This might mean they're less emotional, or maybe it means framing them in a way that gives you an actionable step to dealing with them, or removing any phrases that already specify an outcome.

If some of the statements or judgments are too negative, then don't try to "reframe" it, just write next to the statement, "Instead of judging myself in this way, I could…" and fill in the blank. This will create a trigger for a cognitive disruption, so that every time you do start to judge yourself in that way, you'll remember to change gears, change the channel, and think in a new, more useful way.

Exercise 3

If you have been prone to binging or going off-diet in the past, or simply saying "screw the diet" and going out and having fast food (for example), then try this: Ask yourself, "If that binge or that junk-food meal could talk, what would it be saying to me?"

Once you've answered that question, what does the answer tell you about yourself? Keep the answer in mind the next time you're tempted to go off-diet!

I have observed many clients and former clients who binge eat or sabotage their diet efforts in other ways as well. It is almost always true that you will binge eat or sabotage your diet with foods that you won't really eat *unless* you are specifically trying to sabotage yourself—and this kind of sabotage only happens when you feel really deprived.

The truth is that once you tell your mind that *all* foods are allowed at any time, then foods will lose their allure to your mind and your emotions. You take back the power of "choice." That is a powerful thing to have working for you, instead of telling yourself you have no choice, which tends to work against you. This is all about "right mind" solution.

Further Questions

These questions can be answered as you go. You don't need to answer every one, but I do suggest blocking out some time each week, or every few days, to look at them and consider them.

I've organized them according to which sections of this book they relate to most, so if one section of the book resonated with your more than the others, then by all means, start there!

Introduction and Getting Real

- What does "health" truly mean to you? Have you looked at your weight from the perspective of integrated fitness in the past? How can you look at it in this way in the future?

- Think of a time when you were at your healthiest—just totally on your game. What were the circumstances? What was your disposition? What is different now, or are you there already?

- What are the main sources of stress in your life that you need to be aware of and manage?

- Do you have strategies for coping with stress? Do you sleep more or sleep less? Do you go for walks? Do you have people to whom you can turn?

- What do you do to relax? How often do you do this?

- Do you have structured times for being alone, relaxing, and self-nurturing?

- What is your current relationship status? Do you have a spouse? What emotions surface when you think of this relationship? Is there mutual love and support? Does the relationship itself lift you up and nurture you?

- What aspects of your current lifestyle might affect your weight? Try to list those aspects that are both positive and negative.

- Do you look forward to getting up in the mornings? Why or why not? When is your energy at its highest? What tends to affect your energy most?

Buddha's Eight Steps to End Suffering

- Are you easily distracted and/or do you have trouble sustaining focus on what you consider to be important? (Right focus/right concentration.)

- In general, are you a procrastinator? Do you wait until something "has to be done" before you do it? (Right intention and right action/right behaviour.)

- Do you lack attention to detail? (Right effort and right intention.)

- Do you have trouble with deferred

gratification or with working now for a payoff down the road? (Right intention and right effort.)

- Do you feel restless or calm? (Right mindfulness.)

- Do you get stuck on negative thoughts or do you turn them to positive ones? (Right mindfulness and right perspective.)

- Do you worry excessively? (Right mindfulness, right perspective, and right focus.)

- Do you hold grudges or can you let them go? (Right perspective and right mindfulness.)

Albrecht's Four Mental Habits

- Do you frame your thoughts affirmatively and in useful ways? Try to think of one or two examples.

- Do you see other options in situations? Are you constantly looking for alternative options?

- Make a list of some of the websites,

magazines, reading materials, forums, social networks, and so on that you spend a lot of your time on. Are these places serving you? Which ones are and which ones are not? Be honest. Most people spend time on at least a couple that don't serve them and just invite negative emotions.

- Do you truly value ideas? Can you think of an example where you *did* truly value an idea and an example where you *didn't*? Which one worked out better?

- What are some ideas you've come across recently that it might benefit you to truly value?

- Have you seen diets in the past as only about what is or is not allowed? Can you imagine or entertain a different way of thinking about "the human diet"?

- Have I recently asked myself negative questions like "Why am I such a loser?" or "Why can't I do this?" How did these thoughts serve you or make you feel? Can you rephrase them to be more empowering?

- What options and opportunities are

actually opened up for *you* by taking a more mindful, integrative approach to "dieting"? What new ideas have you recently learned, and what options and opportunities to they present?

Overall Health

- How are your energy levels, and how is this related to your weight issues? Can you identify any patterns with respect to your energy levels? Can you take this into account in structuring your most important activities and/or thinking about times you most tend to do things like snack?

- How is your immune system? Are you sick a lot? Do you feel "under the weather" more often than not? How might this be related to your weight? Research shows that eating healthier is often easier for people if it *really is* for truth "health" and not just to lose weight. Remember, our goal is *integrated* fitness.

- Do you use or abuse tobacco, caffeine, alcohol, pain medications, food, sugar, or other substances? How often and in what quantities? A little bit? More than a little bit? How does the use of these substances affect your life?

Food and Nutrition

- Do you eat slowly or quickly? How many times per day do you eat? Do you have structured meal times?

- Do you savour your meals or do you eat "on the go"?

- Are you always either "on" or "off" a diet? How might this change?

- What are some instances in which you can remember bringing mindful awareness to your eating? When did you savour the foods and also appreciate what they did to and for your body?

- Do you have any specific issues like binging, mindless snacking, or late-night snacking? Brainstorm positive, strategic ways to deal with these. Remember to frame things in an empowering, useful way.

- Do you use health bars, meal replacement

bars, or other "health" foods? Remember, if it has more than five ingredients, it's not *really* a healthy whole food.

Exercise

- What emotions do you feel when you think of "exercise"? Are they positive, negative, neutral? Are your thoughts regarding exercise motivating or demotivating? What does this tell you about your current mindset towards exercise? Again, if it's necessary, can you shift your perspective to one that will truly serve you?

- What kind of exercise do you do right now? Is it cardio-oriented, based on weights and resistance training, or sports-related?

- Think back to a time you really, truly enjoyed exercising. What was it like? Why did you enjoy it? What can you learn from this and apply to your life now?

- Do you prefer to exercise alone or in a group?

- Is exercise truly "built in" to your current

lifestyle, or is it something you try to fit in "here and there" or "when you have the chance"?

- Do you track calories burned during exercise? If so, how might this actually hurt you? Does it add excitement to your routine?

- What kinds of activities bring you joy? What do you look forward to? What aspects of these other activities might be just as applicable to exercise?

Learn More

To learn more about diet, training, and physique transformation, or to get announcements about future books, please visit my website and subscribe to my email list: **http://scottabelfitness.com/**. I send out free articles on nutrition and working out, as well as case studies, client updates, and more.

If you liked this book, and want to see more, please take a moment to **write a review on Amazon** and let me know!

Thank you for purchasing and taking the time to read this book!

ALL RIGHTS RESERVED. No part of this publication may be reproduced or transmitted in any form whatsoever, electronic, or mechanical, including photocopying, recording, or by any informational storage or retrieval system without express written, dated and signed permission from the author.

DISCLAIMER AND/OR LEGAL NOTICES:
Every effort has been made to accurately represent this book and it's potential. Results vary with every individual, and your results may or may not be different from those depicted. No promises, guarantees or warranties, whether stated or implied, have been made that you will produce any specific result from this book. Your efforts are individual and unique, and may vary from those shown. Your success depends on your efforts, background and motivation.

The material in this publication is provided for educational and informational purposes only and is not intended as medical advice. The information contained in this book should not be used to diagnose or treat any illness, metabolic disorder, disease or health problem. Always consult your physician or health care provider before beginning any nutrition or exercise program. Use of the programs, advice, and information contained in this book is at the sole choice and risk of the reader.

Manufactured by Amazon.ca
Acheson, AB